Intuitive Eating for a Balanced Happy Life

food journal & happiness tracker

Kat Zuanich Wellness

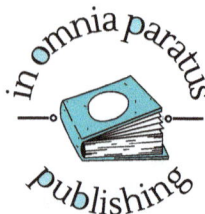

in omnia paratus publishing

Dedication

This journal was created with love for those who have struggled with traditional nutritional habits and diet culture. For those who've spent too much time wondering why nothing stuck or worked. I have so much admiration and empathy for you, and how hard that journey feels.

You are seen. You are appreciated. You are amazing.

I want to send special appreciation to one of my greatest personal inspirations and cheerleaders, my counselor Marguerite Johnson. Thank you for seeing and inspiring me to reach for more love for myself and others. I could never have imagined the confidence and compassion I've attained since you came into my life. Thank you so much.

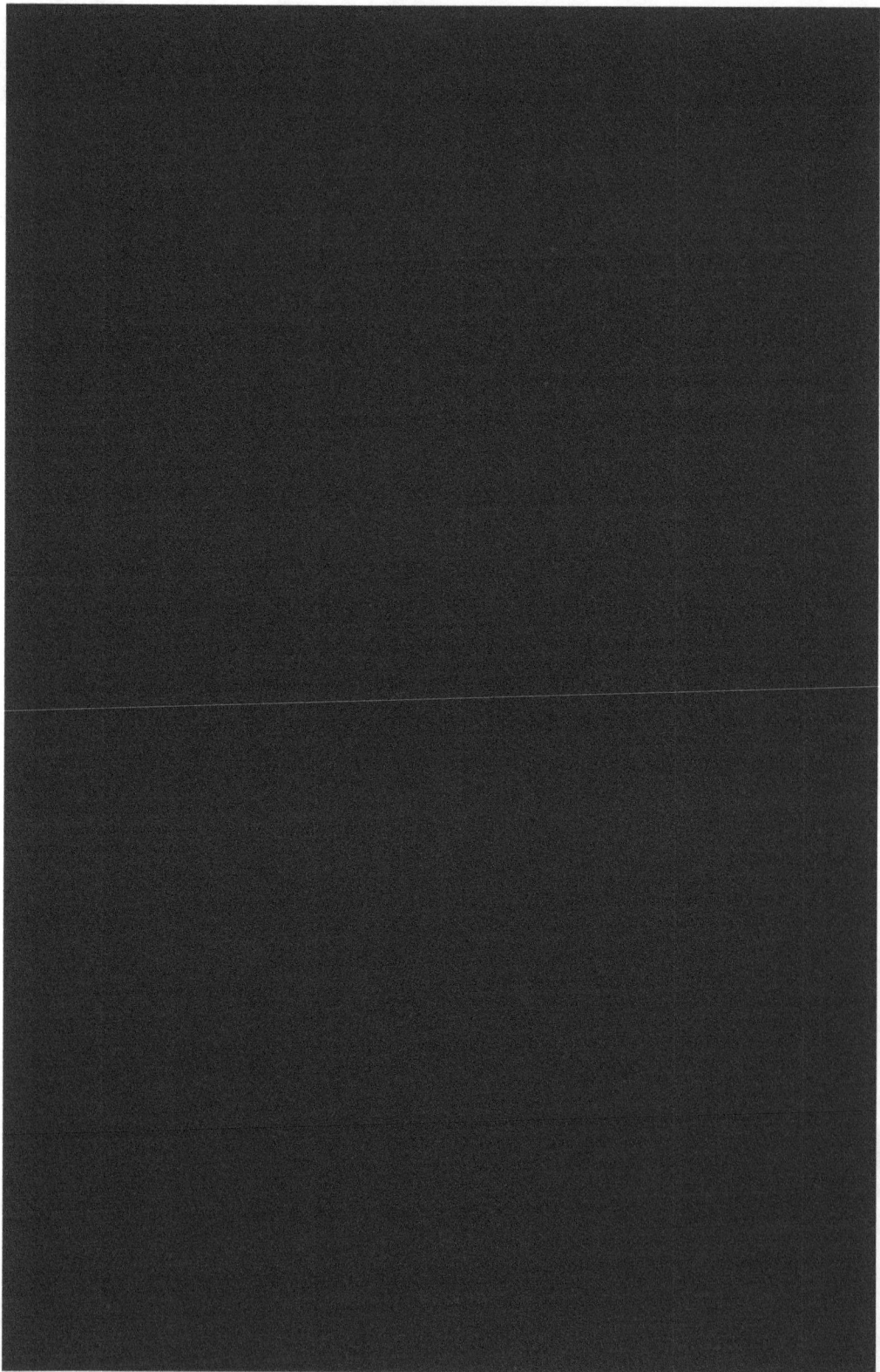

Introduction

Hey new friend!

Congrat's on taking a HUGE step towards claiming your own balanced & happy life through the magic of intuitive eating.

I have tried so many diets that have left me feeling defeated and guilty about perceived failures when those around me have found so much success. There are many healthy lifestyle choices out there, but that does not mean they will work for you and a setback in your goals is only communication from one of your best true norths, which is yourself, that you deserve something different. The one thing, in terms of nutrition, we all deserve is to feel good about the decisions we make and enjoy our lives to the very fullest.

Intuitive eating, in the way I perceive it, can be for everyone on any eating plan and is a tool to learn a mindful approach to what your body is really telling you. It has been such a facilitator of empowerment and self-love in a world that felt harsh and judgmental for me, which has led to a happier weight and a happier life for myself and hopefully for anyone that can push aside the guilt to try it.

So, you may be wondering, who's Kat?

I am a certified personal trainer and chef, currently pursuing my bachelor's degree in wellness management through the University of Wisconsin. I'm incredibly passionate about helping people find confidence and self-appreciation in their health journey.

While I'm still working on my own best-fit healthy lifestyle I believe that through self-compassion and gratitude we can all achieve our own versions of perfect health.

I also believe we can learn more by listening to our own bodies than we can from advice we find on the internet, and that by educating ourselves on a few basic scientific rules, we can better understand why we feel the way we do and make better intuitive choices for ourselves.

Each of us is an incredibly unique being, with unique needs and wants, but as a culture we've been poisoned by the idea that to be worthy we must look, eat, and move in a certain way, ignoring our body's unique mental, physical, developmental, and emotional needs.

For example, I tend to feel better on low animal fat/higher fiber diet (after years of GI and weight problems from Paleo and Low-Carb lifestyles), but after participating in long and strenuous cardiovascular activity (3+ hours), my body responds completely differently and in fact, feels pretty terrible without a boost from healthy animal fats and proteins.

Having been a victim of eating disorders as well as addiction to substances and ideas, based on the countless f'd up fad diets being shouted out in society, I'm on a mission to spread a message of acceptance, mindfulness, and trust in ourselves as perfect works-in-progress.

By increasing our innate sense of what qualifies as nutrient-dense for us as individuals, based on an appreciation, without judgment, of how we feel after eating different foods or beverages, we're able to cultivate maintainable long-term healthy lifestyles as well as a love for our bodies beyond aesthetic ideals.

I always encourage regular participation in physical activities, however to keep things simple there is no specific requirement to track this. It is much simpler to master one technique at a time when it comes to mindfulness, in my opinion, so while in time you will likely find it handy to track exercise in conjunction with nutrition it is not necessary or encouraged at first.

You'll also notice that this journal doesn't include specific areas to track your measurements or weight. While you're welcome to continue tracking those items if you so choose, I've left those pieces out in hopes of allowing you to focus more on eating until you're full and trusting your body to know what that looks and feels like.

This can be difficult at first, especially if you're recovering from obsessive diet practices or a binge-eating habit, but I believe in time you'll rediscover the innate skills we each possess, to recognize our body's unique signs of hunger and satiety, as well as which foods trigger unhealthy energy management.

I also believe that it's less important to track the things we eat and drink in units than it is to recognize how our body feels throughout the eating and drinking process. Instead of feeling guilty about a night on the town with friends, recognize how much your body can handle and in what circumstances, while still maintaining positive energy, focus and mood. Food is more than nutrition; it is culture and a major part of the closeness between humans.

It is perfectly reasonable to get back into a more vigilant nutrition program once this is completed. Intuitive eating is meant to be used solo or as a way to enhance other programs by developing a deeper relationship with our bodies and our food.

Now, to address a few of the most common questions I get asked when it comes to nutrition.

What are Macros?

Macros short for macronutrients are the nutrients found in large amounts, otherwise known as carbohydrates, proteins, and fats. Macronutrients are where the fuel component comes into play but is still quite bio-specific, in my opinion. While in the past many fad diets have involved counting calories, more and more people are recognizing that being mindful of their macro intake can have a much greater impact on their health and well-being than the practice of simply counting and restricting caloric intake.

What are Carbohydrates?

Carbohydrates are the fastest and most readily available form of energy in your body. Carbohydrates consist of sugars, starches, and fibers that all break down through body processes into glucose otherwise known as blood sugar, to supply immediate energy to muscles and organs, or to be stored in the liver for later use. The more complex the carbohydrate the longer it takes to fully break down, which is why different carbohydrates maintain the feeling of fullness and satiety for different lengths of time. They also include dietary fiber, which is key for maintaining healthy pooping habits as well as overall immune function.

What are Proteins?

Proteins are large, complex molecules made up of one or more long chains of amino acids; they regulate and execute almost every function within a cell, and are required for the structure, function, and regulation of the tissues and organs that make up the body. They are essential for the recovery of muscles with exercise, proper enzymatic reactions within cells, proper communication within the body, and many other highly important functions.

What are Fats?

Fats are the most energy-dense macronutrients we consume and are the main component in brain and nervous system formation, maintenance, and growth. DHA Omega-3s found in fatty fish and algae, can also play a major role in mood and other mental acuity issues. Fats are also essential for proper, even energy and hormone health. As with the other two macronutrients (Carbohydrates and Proteins) there are varying types of fats, the main two being saturated and unsaturated. The unsaturated fats are then subdivided into monounsaturated and polyunsaturated. There is nothing inherently 'bad' about any of these natural fats, and there are essential aspects to consuming them all, but the balance is important. The easiest way that I check and regulate my fat ratios is by monitoring only the polyunsaturated fats which should ideally be 1:1 of omega-6 to omega-3 fatty acids. In the modern world, there will be fluctuation to this and that is okay, but if you notice things getting a little too far out of whack it may be worth changing things up.

Omega-3s come primarily from marine, game, or certain plant sources whereas omega-6s are most often consumed in nuts, seeds, eggs, and vegetable oils. The source of the fat is also very important, as the makeup of fatty acids within a food varies greatly depending on the quality of the source. For example, beef that comes from modern 'factory' farming contains significantly fewer polyunsaturated fats by percentage than from cows that were allowed to roam and eat a more traditional and varied diet with ample exercise.

It's my personal and professional belief that if you're going to prioritize one macronutrient to spend a little extra on, this would be the one. Fats comes from many sources that are both animal and plant-based and can be managed easily when you consume ample amounts of both. However, if you prefer to eat only plant-based fats it's perfectly acceptable to get them all from vegetables and nuts alone, maybe supplementing fish oil to maintain a proper balance.

The fats that you should do your best to avoid are trans fats. These come from shortenings and partially hydrogenated oils often, but not always, found in processed foods and some restaurant cooking. While there've been some amazing advances in the processed food brands and options we have available, and there's nothing wrong with convenience, it's important to read the labels of these items, and be aware of what you're choosing to put into your body.

What are Micronutrients?

As the name suggests micronutrients or micros, are the vitamins and minerals found in very small amounts within foods that don't directly produce energy but are essential for daily life and health. Vitamins are either fat-soluble or water-soluble and are organic materials made in plants and animals, while minerals are inorganic and exist in soil and water. These are all essential for proper immune function, growth, brain development and maintenance, proper organ function, and often preventing and fighting disease.

What is Intuitive Eating?

The general principle behind intuitive eating is to understand what you're putting in your system and to pay attention to the obvious effects it has on your energy, mood, and general well-being. Intuitive eating involves a lot of thought and mindfulness about how you feel over time, in different circumstances, in your gut and mental health. It tends to be a slow or even stagnant path to weight loss, at least at first, but once your body discovers and settles into the right rhythm you can quickly achieve a perfect balance of weight, life, and health.

I personally choose to follow an intuitive eating pattern, which is the basis of this journal & tracker. While I understand that for many people, the idea of intuitive eating can seem too 'general' or 'unstructured,' I think it's important to recognize the ways in which our bodies communicate with us, regarding what they need more of, less of, and what leaves us feeling healthiest and happiest.

On the next few pages, I've provided sample daily tracker pages showing some of my own daily choices, feelings, and realizations.

A few of the key points I've realized through my own tracking are:

- There are parts of meals that seem to trigger negative feelings for me.
- There are other parts of meals that seem to make me feel good.
- Although I love coffee, my body does much better with lower-acid versions like cold brew or espresso, over drip, and sometimes black tea is a better bet altogether.

Keep in mind as you review these sample pages, and begin your own tracking, that there is no wrong way to go about this practice. The goal is to know yourself better, strengthening the connection you have with your body, what it needs, wants, and doesn't.

It takes time to see the patterns of our eating that aren't working for us, but with time, I believe anyone can optimize what works best for them. It's when we adopt and embrace intuitive habits that long-term, life-enriching changes occur.

Ready to get started? Let's go!

DATE   May 15, 2022   (S) M T W T F S

MORNING THOUGHTS & FEELINGS

Woke up before my alarm, feeling energized despite only sleeping 6.5
hours; had a fun day planned of work I enjoy, sunshine and a hike with my
pup and a friend.

MORNING MEAL @ ___6:30am___

I ATE:
steel cut oats, sliced strawberries & banana, whole fat greek yogurt, maple
syrup, mixed nut butter, cinnamon & vanilla extract

I DRANK:
water & black coffee

I FELT:
full, energized, slight stomach ache

2-3 HOURS LATER I FELT:
full, really steady energy

MID MORNING SNACK @ ___9:30am___

I ATE:
nothing

I DRANK:
water & kombucha

I FELT:
full from breakfast, slightly antsy

AFTERNOON MEAL @   2:00pm

I ATE:

sharp cheddar cheese, triscuit crackers, granny smith apple

I DRANK:

IPA Beer

I FELT:

slightly buzzed, a little dehydrated, decent energy level

2-3 HOURS LATER I FELT:

satisfied enough, a little irritable

AFTERNOON SNACK @   N/A

I ATE:

nothing

I DRANK:

nothing

I FELT:

full-enough, still a little tired and irritable

EVENING MEAL @   7:00pm

I ATE:

Grass-fed beef burger with pepperjack, jalapenos, mayo, bbq sauce &
veggies, no bun, sweet potato oven-fries with spicy aioli, green salad w/
tomatoes, carrots, radish and pepitas; balsamic vinaigrette

I DRANK:

2 glasses of wine (while cooking) & water

I FELT:

very full, but not bloated, ready for bed, relaxed

2-3 HOURS LATER I FELT:

in bed, tired, relaxed, happy

HAPPINESS TRACKER - ON A SCALE OF 1-5

Rate the areas below from 1-5, with 1 being least happy & 5 being most happy. Pay close attention to any trends you begin to notice regarding how the things you eat & drink affect the way you feel & your overall happiness.

	Rating
My morning energy level	● ● ● ● ○
My afternoon energy level	● ● ● ○ ○
My evening energy level	● ● ○ ○ ○
How my body feels	● ● ● ○ ○
My mental clarity	● ● ● ● ○
My emotional stability	● ● ● ● ○
My excitement about life	● ● ● ● ○
My personal relationships	● ● ● ○ ○
My professional relationships	● ● ● ○ ○
My poop	● ● ● ○ ○

EVENING THOUGHTS & FEELINGS

_____

_____

_____

_____

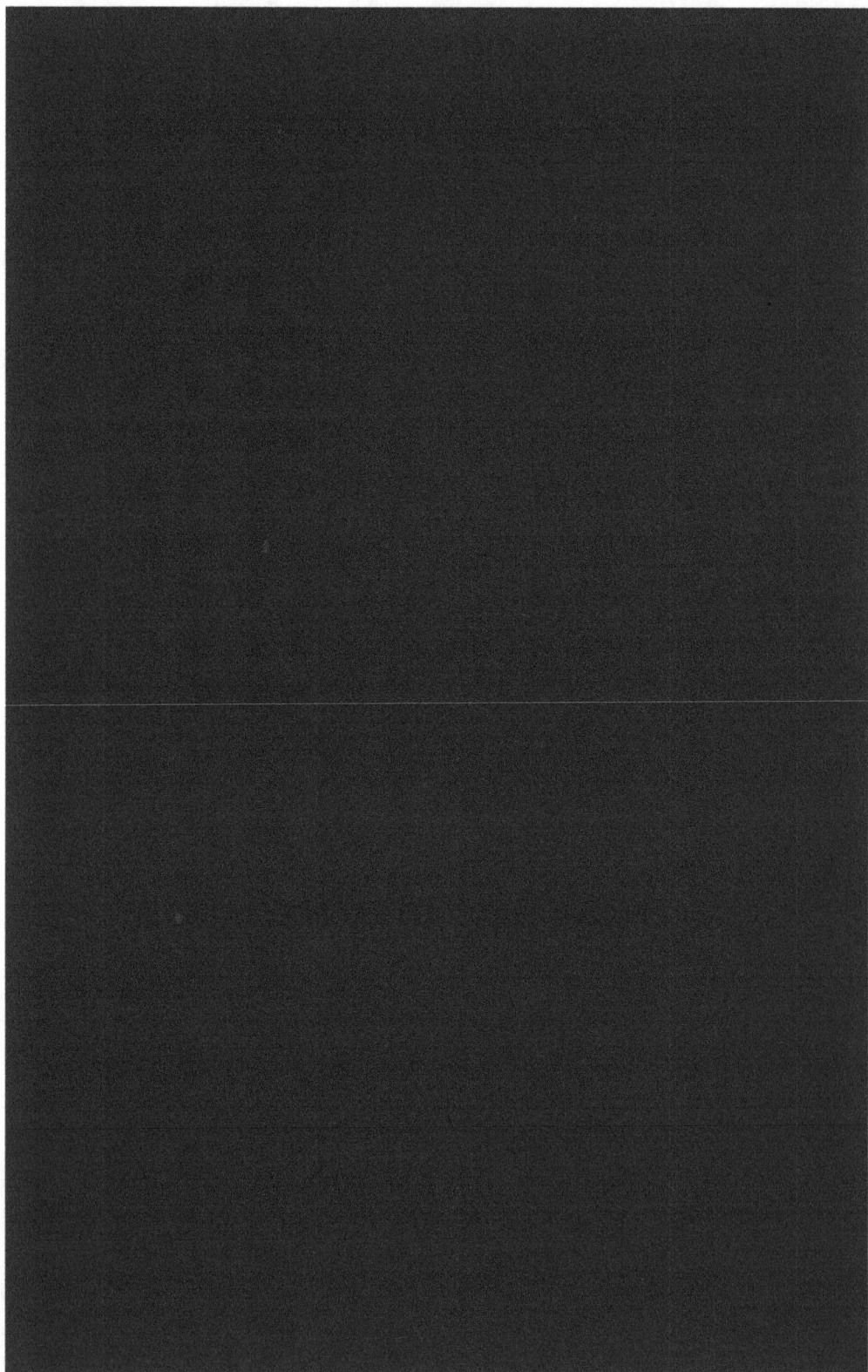

DATE May 16, 2022   S (M) T W T F S

MORNING THOUGHTS & FEELINGS

I woke up to my alarm, a little tired still because my dog kept waking me up. I was under some internal pressure to accomplish a lot for the day, but I meditated and calmed my insecurities.

MORNING MEAL @ _____ 6:00am

I ATE:

eggs scrambled, corn tortillas, piece of bacon, butter, salsa verde, pickled red cabbage

I DRANK:

1 pint water & 2 cups black coffee

I FELT:

congested, full, energized, slightly nauseous

2-3 HOURS LATER I FELT:

hungry again, upset stomach, and diarrhea

MID MORNING SNACK @ _____ 10:00am

I ATE:

honeycrisp apple, mixed nut butter

I DRANK:

water & kombucha

I FELT:

satisfied, stomach settled, full

AFTERNOON MEAL @   1:30pm

I ATE:

vegan chocolate protein powder, full fat greek yogurt, frozen cherries, banana, mushroom complex powder, cinnamon

I DRANK:

sparkling water & green juice

I FELT:

not super full, but not hungry, energized, strong

2-3 HOURS LATER I FELT:

craving sugar or caffeine, a little snacky and withdrawn

AFTERNOON SNACK @   4:00pm

I ATE:

chocolate chips, whole grain toast, almond butter

I DRANK:

iced tea

I FELT:

picked up, but still less focused on work than I was hoping and goofier

EVENING MEAL @   7:00pm

I ATE:

spicy chickpea and paneer curry with lots of veggies, basmati rice, kimchee, gluten-free, dairy-free chocolate chip macadamia nut cookie

I DRANK:

sparkling water & chamomile tea

I FELT:

very nourished, full, sleepy

2-3 HOURS LATER I FELT:

in bed, tired, relaxed, happy

HAPPINESS TRACKER - ON A SCALE OF 1-5

Rate the areas below from 1-5, with 1 being least happy & 5 being most happy. Pay close attention to any trends you begin to notice regarding how the things you eat & drink affect the way you feel & your overall happiness.

My morning energy level ● ● ● ● ○

My afternoon energy level ● ● ● ○ ○

My evening energy level ● ● ○ ○ ○

How my body feels ● ● ● ○ ○

My mental clarity ● ● ● ● ○

My emotional stability ● ● ● ● ○

My excitement about life ● ● ● ● ○

My personal relationships ● ● ● ○ ○

My professional relationships ● ● ● ○ ○

My poop ● ● ● ○ ○

EVENING THOUGHTS & FEELINGS

_____

_____

_____

_____

DATE   May 17, 2022   S M (T) W T F S

MORNING THOUGHTS & FEELINGS

Woke up a little before my alarm, but still tired, lots to do before a
bachelorette party and road trip, meditated for grounding.

MORNING MEAL @ _____ 7:00am _____

I ATE:

jalapeno bagel with cream cheese, poached eggs, tomato, red onion, sprouts

I DRANK:

hot black tea & green juice

I FELT:

still a little tired, but more grounded & satisfied, no stomach discomfort at all

2-3 HOURS LATER I FELT:

good, stressed about school, knowing I would be gone for a couple of nights

MID MORNING SNACK @ _____ 10:00am _____

I ATE:

nothing

I DRANK:

water

I FELT:

I don't have the best appetite when I'm focused especially after taking
ADHD medication; I was getting a lot done though so my stress was eased

AFTERNOON MEAL @ ___1:00pm___

I ATE:

vegan chocolate protein shake, whole fat greek yogurt, spinach, mixed nut
butter, banana, cinnamon, mushroom complex powder, whole grain crackers
chevre, tomatoes

I DRANK:

sparkling water

I FELT:

nourished, focused, a little antsy to leave

2-3 HOURS LATER I FELT:

AFTERNOON SNACK @ ___4:00pm___

I ATE:

some charcuterie at a bar

I DRANK:

1 glass champagne, 1 shot reposado tequila, sparkling water

I FELT:

buzzed, joyful, silly - 2 hours later: hungry, loopy, happy

EVENING MEAL @ 7:00 - 10:00pm

I ATE:

carnitas tacos, rice, beans, guacamole and salsas

I DRANK:

2 tequila sodas, 2 light beers, 1 shot reposado tequila

I FELT:

drunk, very silly, very friendly and affectionate

2-3 HOURS LATER I FELT:

tired and in bed, groggy, but still silly and filled with love

HAPPINESS TRACKER - ON A SCALE OF 1-5

Rate the areas below from 1-5, with 1 being least happy & 5 being most happy. Pay close attention to any trends you begin to notice regarding how the things you eat & drink affect the way you feel & your overall happiness.

My morning energy level	● ● ● ● ○
My afternoon energy level	● ● ● ○ ○
My evening energy level	● ● ○ ○ ○
How my body feels	● ● ● ○ ○
My mental clarity	● ● ● ● ○
My emotional stability	● ● ● ● ○
My excitement about life	● ● ● ● ○
My personal relationships	● ● ● ○ ○
My professional relationships	● ● ● ○ ○
My poop	● ● ● ○ ○

EVENING THOUGHTS & FEELINGS

_____

_____

_____

_____

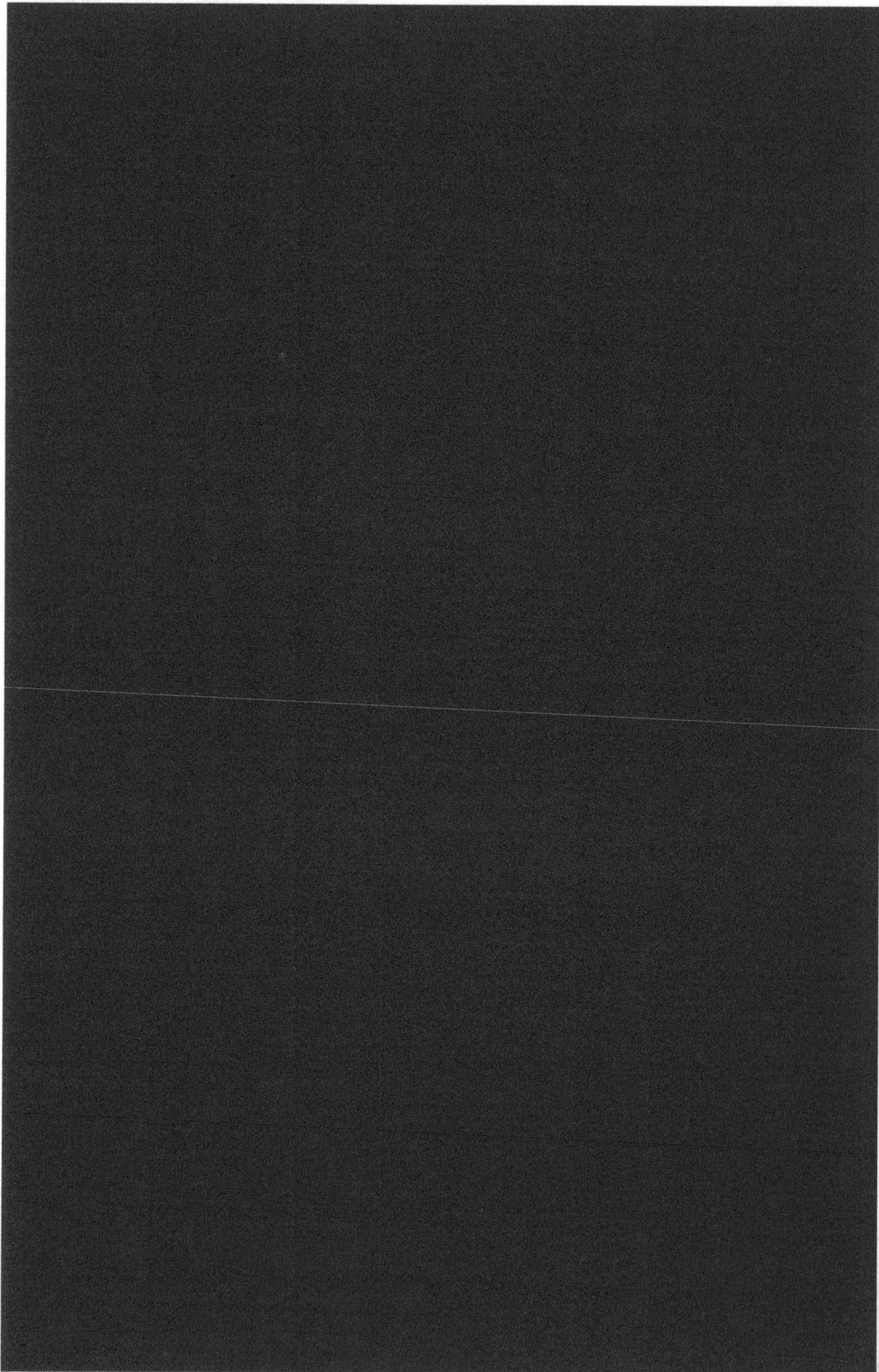

Now it's your turn!

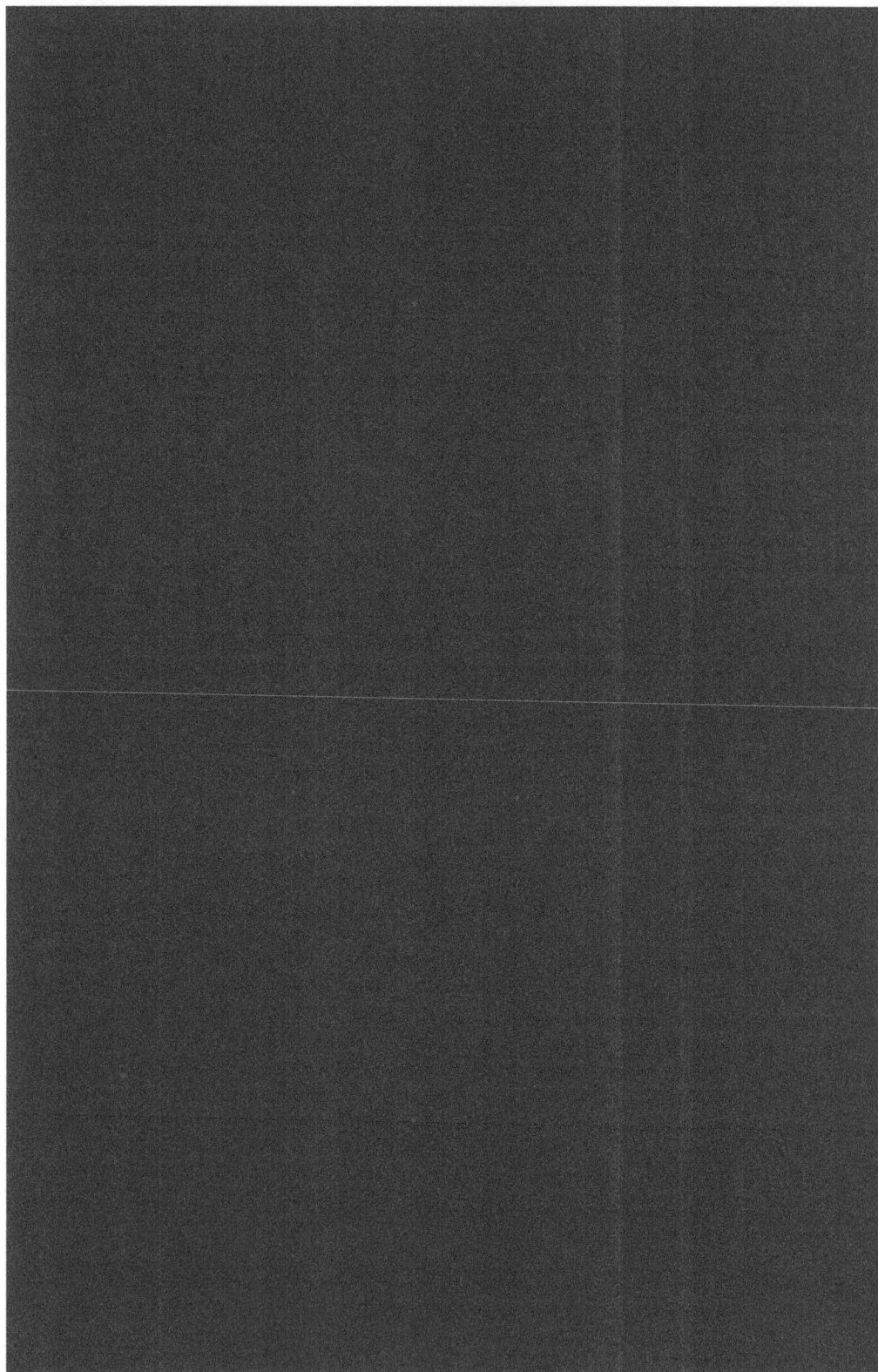

DATE   **S   M   T   W   T   F   S**

MORNING THOUGHTS & FEELINGS

_____
_____
_____
_____
_____

MORNING MEAL @ _____

I ATE:
_____
_____

I DRANK:
_____

I FELT:
_____

2-3 HOURS LATER I FELT:
_____

MID MORNING SNACK @ _____

I ATE:
_____
_____

I DRANK:
_____

I FELT:
_____

AFTERNOON MEAL @ _____

I ATE:

_____

_____

I DRANK:

_____

I FELT:

_____

2-3 HOURS LATER I FELT:

_____

AFTERNOON SNACK @ _____

I ATE:

_____

_____

I DRANK:

_____

I FELT:

_____

EVENING MEAL @ _____

I ATE:

_____

_____

I DRANK:

_____

I FELT:

_____

2-3 HOURS LATER I FELT:

_____

HAPPINESS TRACKER - ON A SCALE OF 1-5

Rate the areas below from 1-5, with 1 being least happy & 5 being most happy. Pay close attention to any trends you begin to notice regarding how the things you eat & drink affect the way you feel & your overall happiness.

My morning energy level   ◯ ◯ ◯ ◯ ◯

My afternoon energy level   ◯ ◯ ◯ ◯ ◯

My evening energy level   ◯ ◯ ◯ ◯ ◯

How my body feels   ◯ ◯ ◯ ◯ ◯

My mental clarity   ◯ ◯ ◯ ◯ ◯

My emotional stability   ◯ ◯ ◯ ◯ ◯

My excitement about life   ◯ ◯ ◯ ◯ ◯

My personal relationships   ◯ ◯ ◯ ◯ ◯

My professional relationships   ◯ ◯ ◯ ◯ ◯

My poop   ◯ ◯ ◯ ◯ ◯

EVENING THOUGHTS & FEELINGS

_____

_____

_____

_____

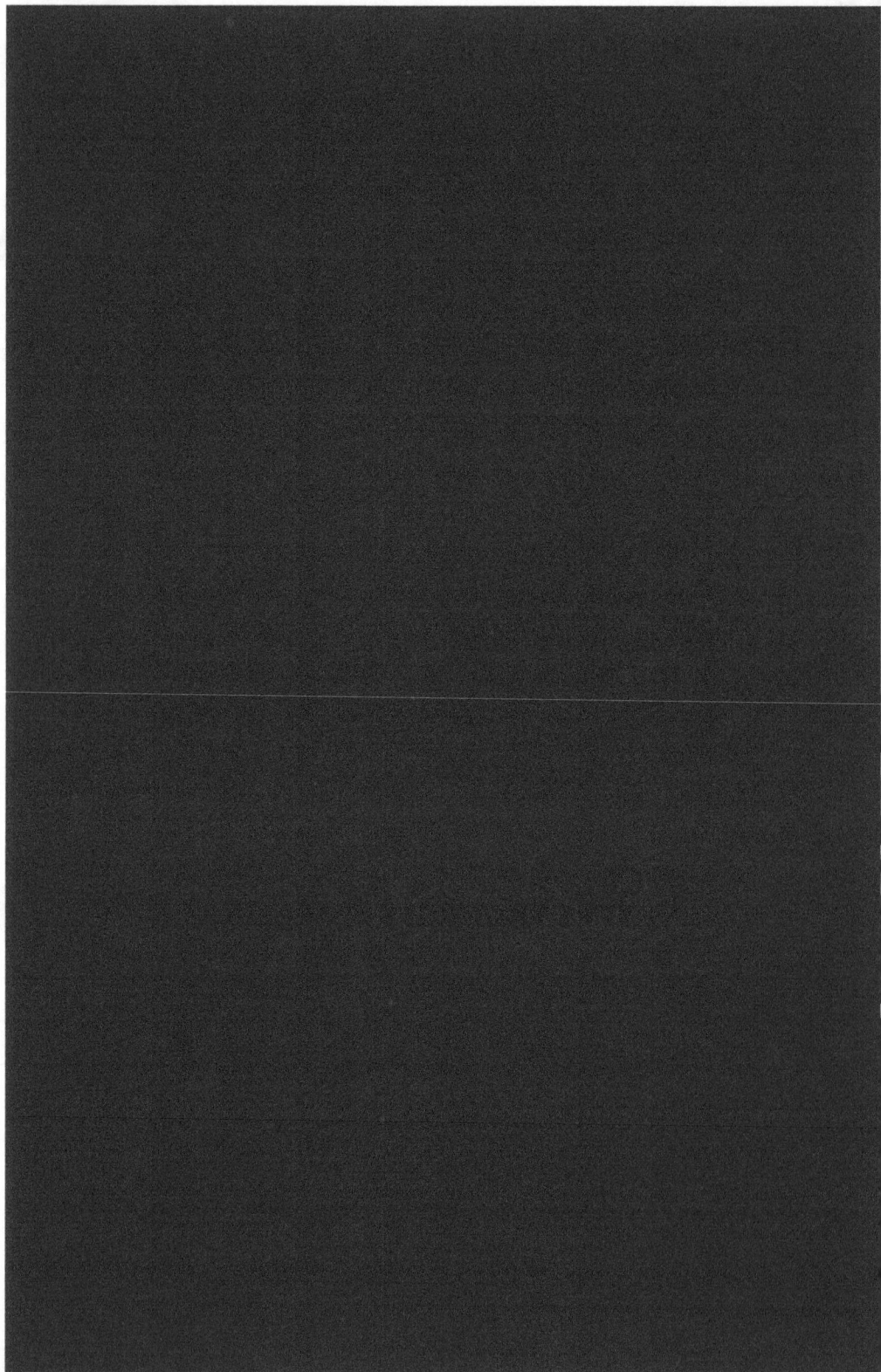

DATE   **S   M   T   W   T   F   S**

MORNING THOUGHTS & FEELINGS

_____

_____

_____

_____

MORNING MEAL @ _____

I ATE:

_____

I DRANK:

_____

I FELT:

_____

2-3 HOURS LATER I FELT:

_____

MID MORNING SNACK @ _____

I ATE:

_____

I DRANK:

_____

I FELT:

_____

AFTERNOON MEAL @ _____

I ATE:

_____
_____

I DRANK:

_____

I FELT:

_____

2-3 HOURS LATER I FELT:

_____

AFTERNOON SNACK @ _____

I ATE:

_____
_____

I DRANK:

_____

I FELT:

_____

EVENING MEAL @ _____

I ATE:

_____
_____

I DRANK:

_____

I FELT:

_____

2-3 HOURS LATER I FELT:

_____

HAPPINESS TRACKER - ON A SCALE OF 1-5

Rate the areas below from 1-5, with 1 being least happy & 5 being most happy. Pay close attention to any trends you begin to notice regarding how the things you eat & drink affect the way you feel & your overall happiness.

My morning energy level ○ ○ ○ ○ ○

My afternoon energy level ○ ○ ○ ○ ○

My evening energy level ○ ○ ○ ○ ○

How my body feels ○ ○ ○ ○ ○

My mental clarity ○ ○ ○ ○ ○

My emotional stability ○ ○ ○ ○ ○

My excitement about life ○ ○ ○ ○ ○

My personal relationships ○ ○ ○ ○ ○

My professional relationships ○ ○ ○ ○ ○

My poop ○ ○ ○ ○ ○

EVENING THOUGHTS & FEELINGS

_____

_____

_____

_____

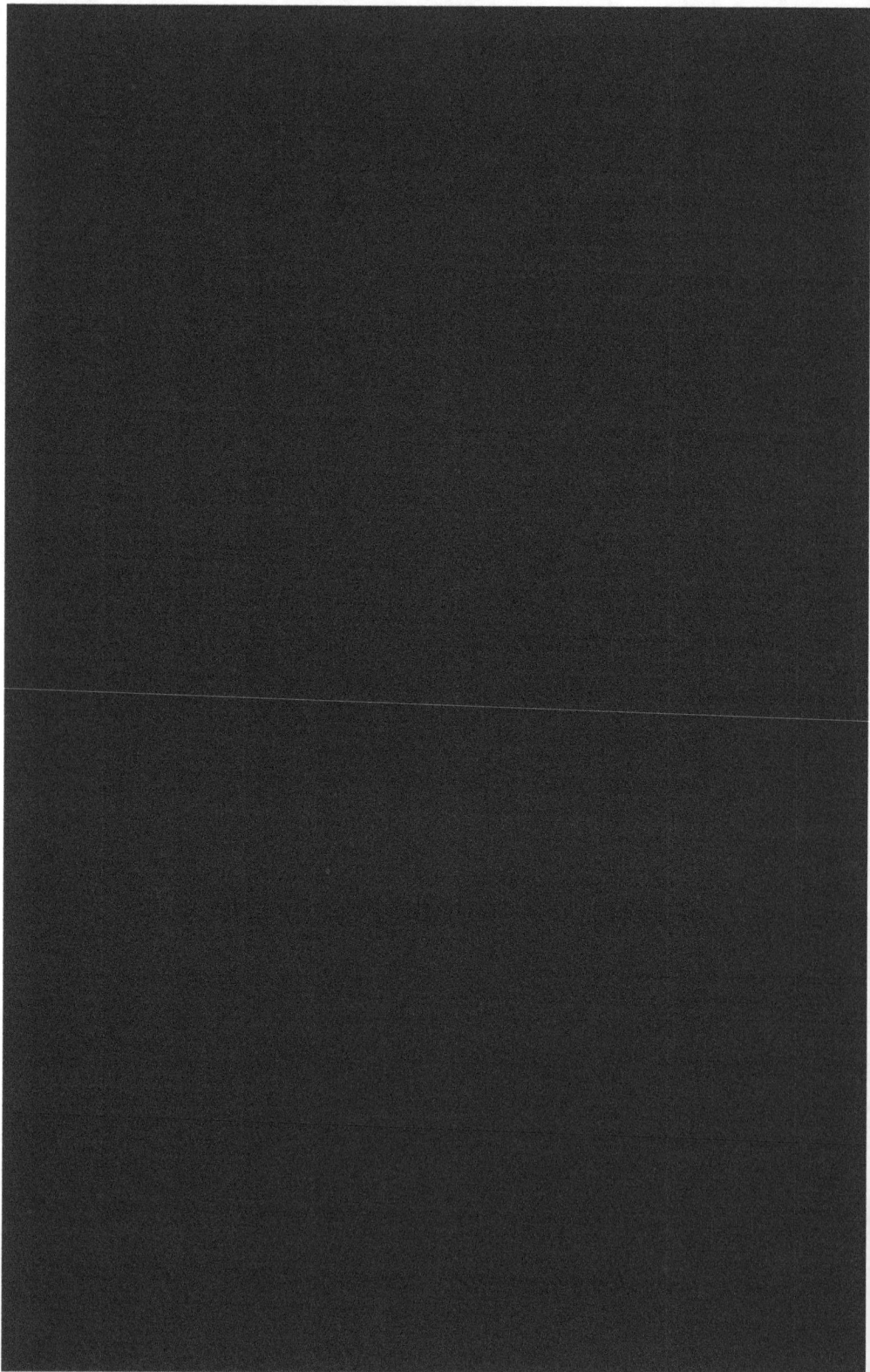

DATE _____ **S M T W T F S**

MORNING THOUGHTS & FEELINGS

_____
_____
_____
_____

MORNING MEAL @ _____

I ATE:
_____
_____

I DRANK:
_____

I FELT:
_____

2-3 HOURS LATER I FELT:
_____

MID MORNING SNACK @ _____

I ATE:
_____
_____

I DRANK:
_____

I FELT:
_____

AFTERNOON MEAL @ _____

I ATE:

_____

_____

I DRANK:

_____

I FELT:

_____

2-3 HOURS LATER I FELT:

_____

AFTERNOON SNACK @ _____

I ATE:

_____

_____

I DRANK:

_____

I FELT:

_____

EVENING MEAL @ _____

I ATE:

_____

_____

I DRANK:

_____

I FELT:

_____

2-3 HOURS LATER I FELT:

_____

HAPPINESS TRACKER - ON A SCALE OF 1-5

Rate the areas below from 1-5, with 1 being least happy & 5 being most happy. Pay close attention to any trends you begin to notice regarding how the things you eat & drink affect the way you feel & your overall happiness.

My morning energy level   ○ ○ ○ ○ ○

My afternoon energy level   ○ ○ ○ ○ ○

My evening energy level   ○ ○ ○ ○ ○

How my body feels   ○ ○ ○ ○ ○

My mental clarity   ○ ○ ○ ○ ○

My emotional stability   ○ ○ ○ ○ ○

My excitement about life   ○ ○ ○ ○ ○

My personal relationships   ○ ○ ○ ○ ○

My professional relationships   ○ ○ ○ ○ ○

My poop   ○ ○ ○ ○ ○

EVENING THOUGHTS & FEELINGS

_____

_____

_____

_____

DATE   **S M T W T F S**

MORNING THOUGHTS & FEELINGS

_____
_____
_____
_____

MORNING MEAL @ _____

I ATE:

_____
_____

I DRANK:

_____

I FELT:

_____

2-3 HOURS LATER I FELT:

_____

MID MORNING SNACK @ _____

I ATE:

_____
_____

I DRANK:

_____

I FELT:

_____

AFTERNOON MEAL @ _____

I ATE:

_____
_____

I DRANK:

_____

I FELT:

_____

2-3 HOURS LATER I FELT:

_____

AFTERNOON SNACK @ _____

I ATE:

_____
_____

I DRANK:

_____

I FELT:

_____

EVENING MEAL @ _____

I ATE:

_____
_____

I DRANK:

_____

I FELT:

_____

2-3 HOURS LATER I FELT:

_____

HAPPINESS TRACKER - ON A SCALE OF 1-5

Rate the areas below from 1-5, with 1 being least happy & 5 being most happy. Pay close attention to any trends you begin to notice regarding how the things you eat & drink affect the way you feel & your overall happiness.

My morning energy level ○ ○ ○ ○ ○

My afternoon energy level ○ ○ ○ ○ ○

My evening energy level ○ ○ ○ ○ ○

How my body feels ○ ○ ○ ○ ○

My mental clarity ○ ○ ○ ○ ○

My emotional stability ○ ○ ○ ○ ○

My excitement about life ○ ○ ○ ○ ○

My personal relationships ○ ○ ○ ○ ○

My professional relationships ○ ○ ○ ○ ○

My poop ○ ○ ○ ○ ○

EVENING THOUGHTS & FEELINGS

_____

_____

_____

_____

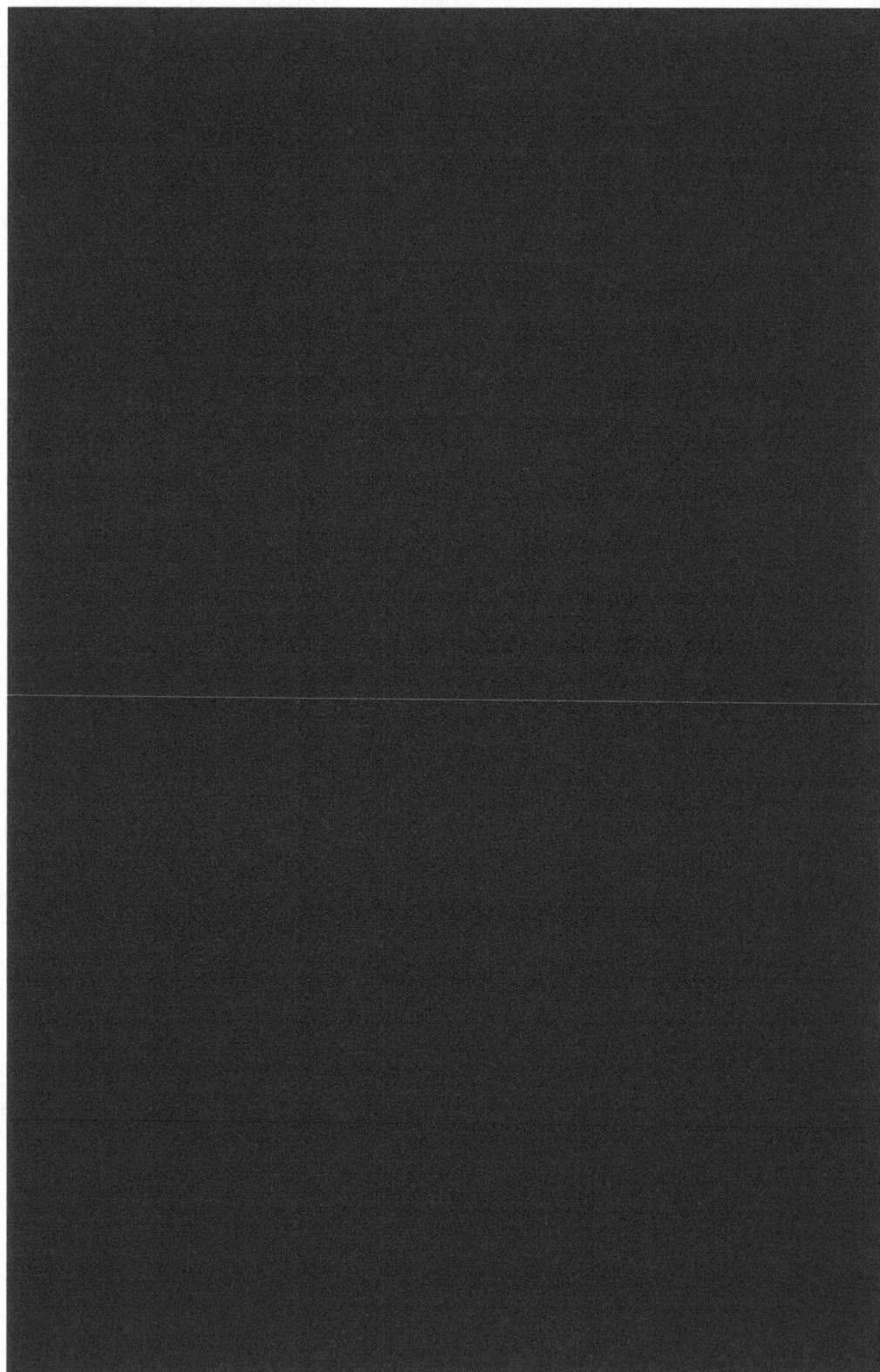

Day 5

DATE   S   M   T   W   T   F   S

MORNING THOUGHTS & FEELINGS

_____

_____

_____

_____

MORNING MEAL @ _____

I ATE:

_____

_____

I DRANK:

_____

I FELT:

_____

2-3 HOURS LATER I FELT:

_____

MID MORNING SNACK @ _____

I ATE:

_____

_____

I DRANK:

_____

I FELT:

_____

AFTERNOON MEAL @ _____

I ATE:

_____

_____

I DRANK:

_____

I FELT:

_____

2-3 HOURS LATER I FELT:

_____

AFTERNOON SNACK @ _____

I ATE:

_____

_____

I DRANK:

_____

I FELT:

_____

EVENING MEAL @ _____

I ATE:

_____

_____

I DRANK:

_____

I FELT:

_____

2-3 HOURS LATER I FELT:

_____

HAPPINESS TRACKER - ON A SCALE OF 1-5

Rate the areas below from 1-5, with 1 being least happy & 5 being most happy. Pay close attention to any trends you begin to notice regarding how the things you eat & drink affect the way you feel & your overall happiness.

My morning energy level   ○ ○ ○ ○ ○

My afternoon energy level   ○ ○ ○ ○ ○

My evening energy level   ○ ○ ○ ○ ○

How my body feels   ○ ○ ○ ○ ○

My mental clarity   ○ ○ ○ ○ ○

My emotional stability   ○ ○ ○ ○ ○

My excitement about life   ○ ○ ○ ○ ○

My personal relationships   ○ ○ ○ ○ ○

My professional relationships   ○ ○ ○ ○ ○

My poop   ○ ○ ○ ○ ○

EVENING THOUGHTS & FEELINGS

_____

_____

_____

_____

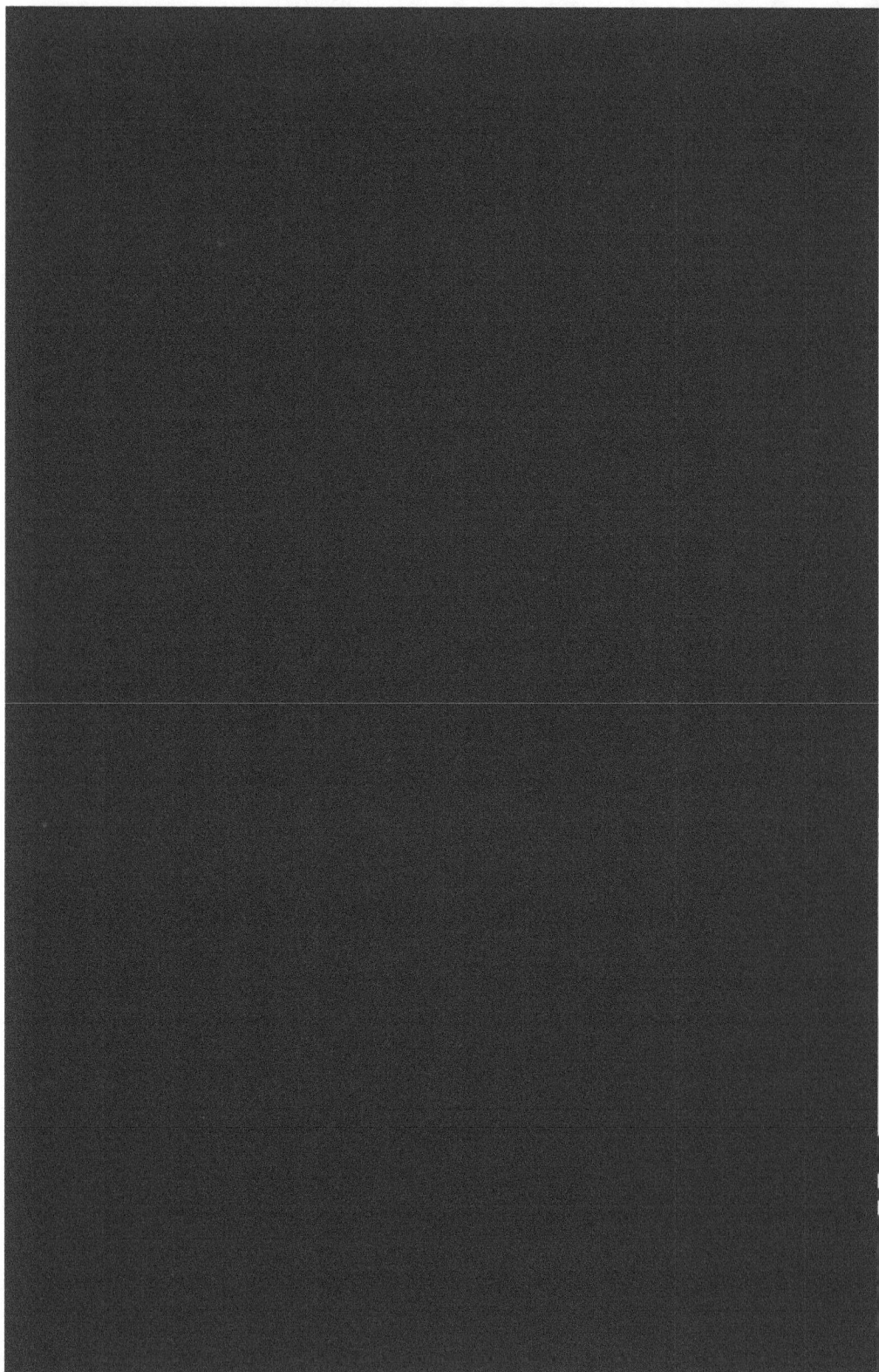

Day 6

DATE   S M T W T F S

MORNING THOUGHTS & FEELINGS

_____
_____
_____
_____

MORNING MEAL @ _____

I ATE:
_____
_____

I DRANK:
_____

I FELT:

2-3 HOURS LATER I FELT:
_____

MID MORNING SNACK @ _____

I ATE:
_____
_____

I DRANK:
_____

I FELT:
_____

AFTERNOON MEAL @ _____

I ATE:

_____
_____

I DRANK:

_____

I FELT:

_____

2-3 HOURS LATER I FELT:

_____

AFTERNOON SNACK @ _____

I ATE:

_____
_____

I DRANK:

_____

I FELT:

_____

EVENING MEAL @ _____

I ATE:

_____
_____

I DRANK:

_____

I FELT:

_____

2-3 HOURS LATER I FELT:

_____

HAPPINESS TRACKER - ON A SCALE OF 1-5

Rate the areas below from 1-5, with 1 being least happy & 5 being most happy. Pay close attention to any trends you begin to notice regarding how the things you eat & drink affect the way you feel & your overall happiness.

My morning energy level	○ ○ ○ ○ ○
My afternoon energy level	○ ○ ○ ○ ○
My evening energy level	○ ○ ○ ○ ○
How my body feels	○ ○ ○ ○ ○
My mental clarity	○ ○ ○ ○ ○
My emotional stability	○ ○ ○ ○ ○
My excitement about life	○ ○ ○ ○ ○
My personal relationships	○ ○ ○ ○ ○
My professional relationships	○ ○ ○ ○ ○
My poop	○ ○ ○ ○ ○

EVENING THOUGHTS & FEELINGS

_____

_____

_____

_____

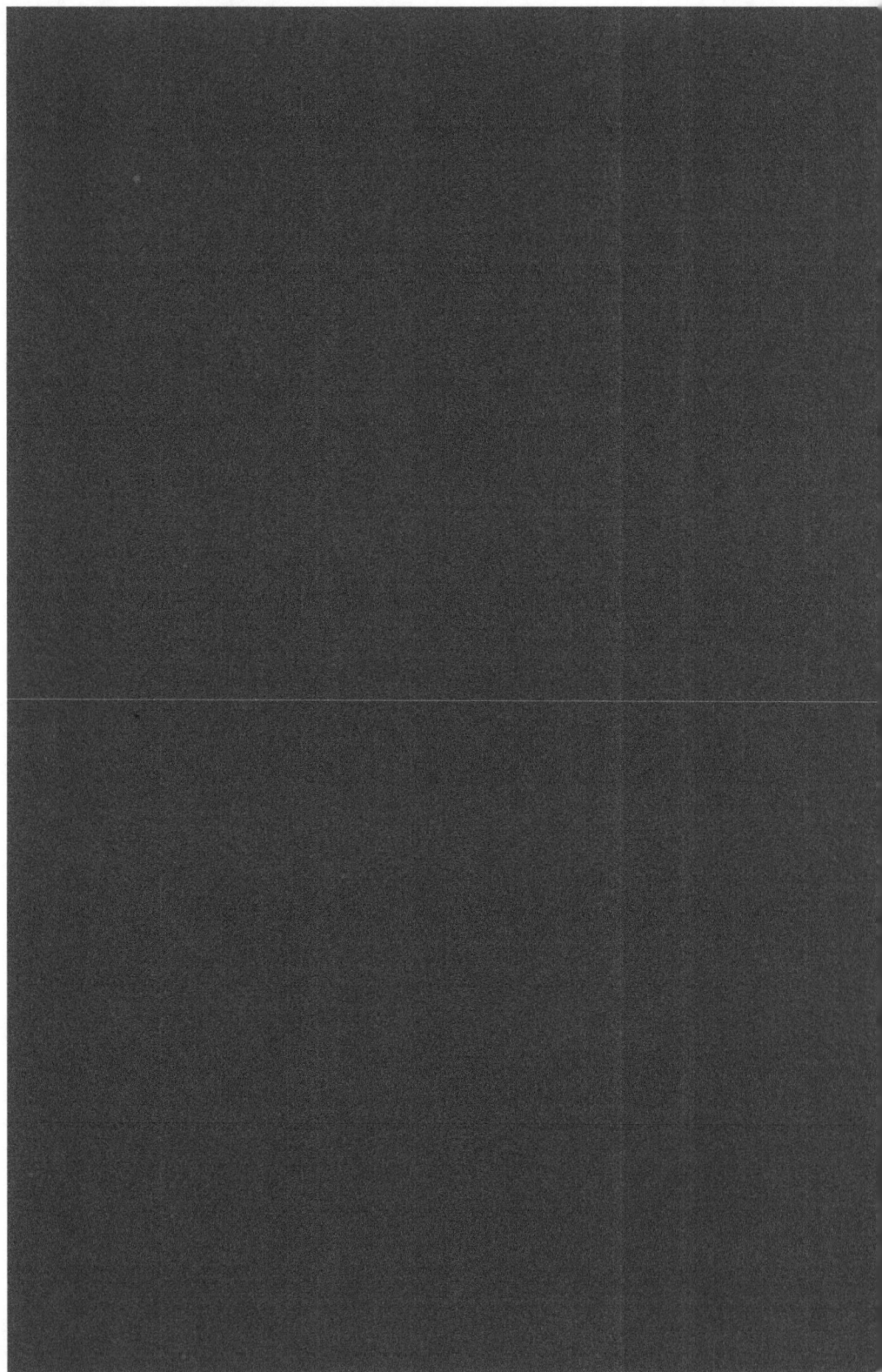

DATE   **S M T W T F S**

MORNING THOUGHTS & FEELINGS

_____
_____
_____
_____

MORNING MEAL @ _____

I ATE:
_____
_____

I DRANK:
_____

I FELT:
_____

2-3 HOURS LATER I FELT:
_____

MID MORNING SNACK @ _____

I ATE:
_____
_____

I DRANK:
_____

I FELT:
_____

AFTERNOON MEAL @ _____

I ATE:

_____
_____

I DRANK:

_____

I FELT:

_____

2-3 HOURS LATER I FELT:

_____

AFTERNOON SNACK @ _____

I ATE:

_____
_____

I DRANK:

_____

I FELT:

_____

EVENING MEAL @ _____

I ATE:

_____
_____

I DRANK:

_____

I FELT:

_____

2-3 HOURS LATER I FELT:

_____

HAPPINESS TRACKER - ON A SCALE OF 1-5

Rate the areas below from 1-5, with 1 being least happy & 5 being most happy. Pay close attention to any trends you begin to notice regarding how the things you eat & drink affect the way you feel & your overall happiness.

My morning energy level ⚪ ⚪ ⚪ ⚪ ⚪

My afternoon energy level ⚪ ⚪ ⚪ ⚪ ⚪

My evening energy level ⚪ ⚪ ⚪ ⚪ ⚪

How my body feels ⚪ ⚪ ⚪ ⚪ ⚪

My mental clarity ⚪ ⚪ ⚪ ⚪ ⚪

My emotional stability ⚪ ⚪ ⚪ ⚪ ⚪

My excitement about life ⚪ ⚪ ⚪ ⚪ ⚪

My personal relationships ⚪ ⚪ ⚪ ⚪ ⚪

My professional relationships ⚪ ⚪ ⚪ ⚪ ⚪

My poop ⚪ ⚪ ⚪ ⚪ ⚪

EVENING THOUGHTS & FEELINGS

_____

_____

_____

_____

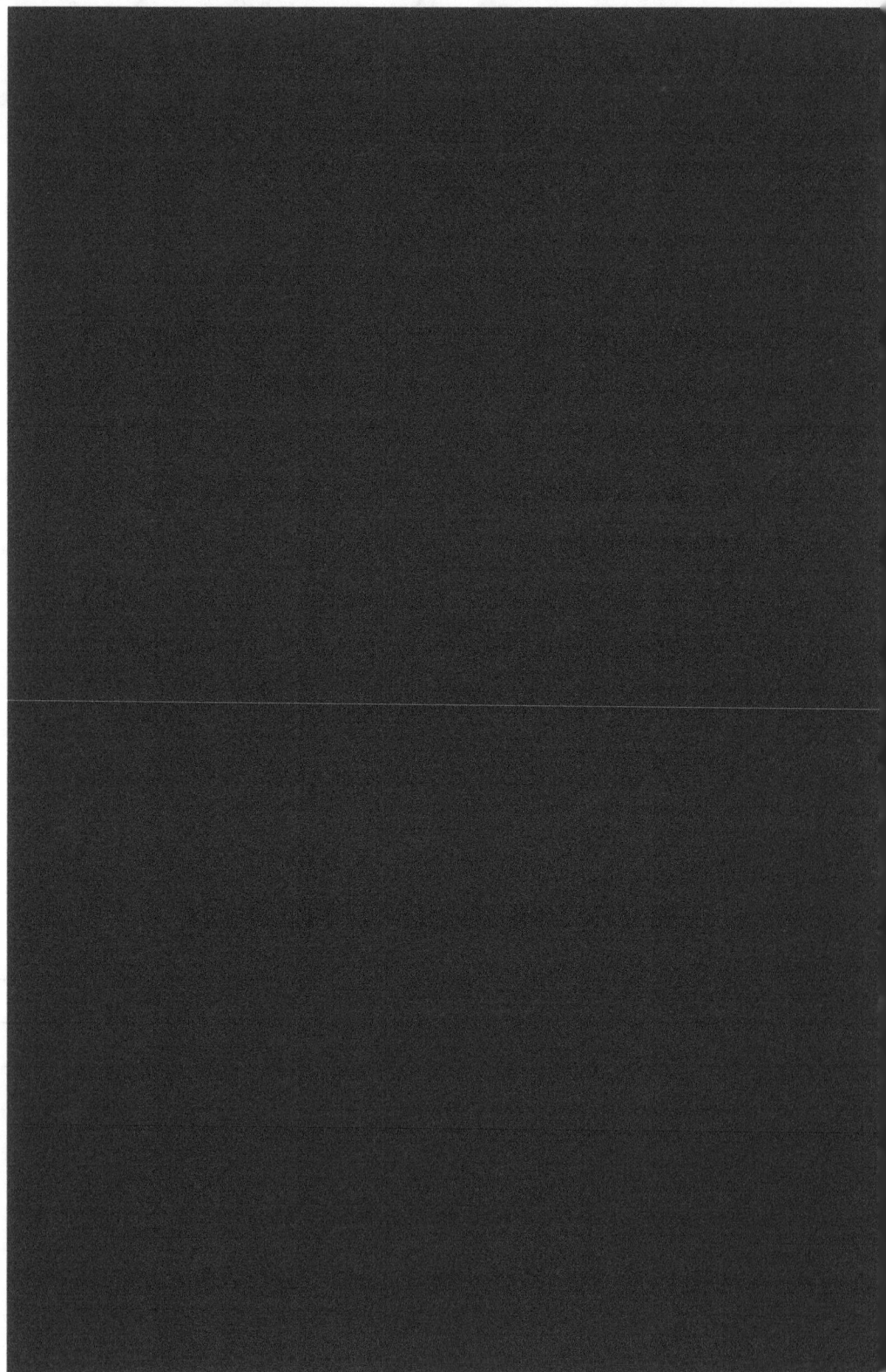

Well done!

Time flies when you're having fun & living a balanced life - you've been eating intuitively & tracking your happiness for a full week already.

Have you noticed any trends in what you're eating & how you're feeling?

It's important to recognize & appreciate the amazing progress you're making every single day.

How are you treating yourself?

Whether your idea of self-care is a massage, pedicure, seeing a movie or taking a trip to the bookstore - Treat yourself!

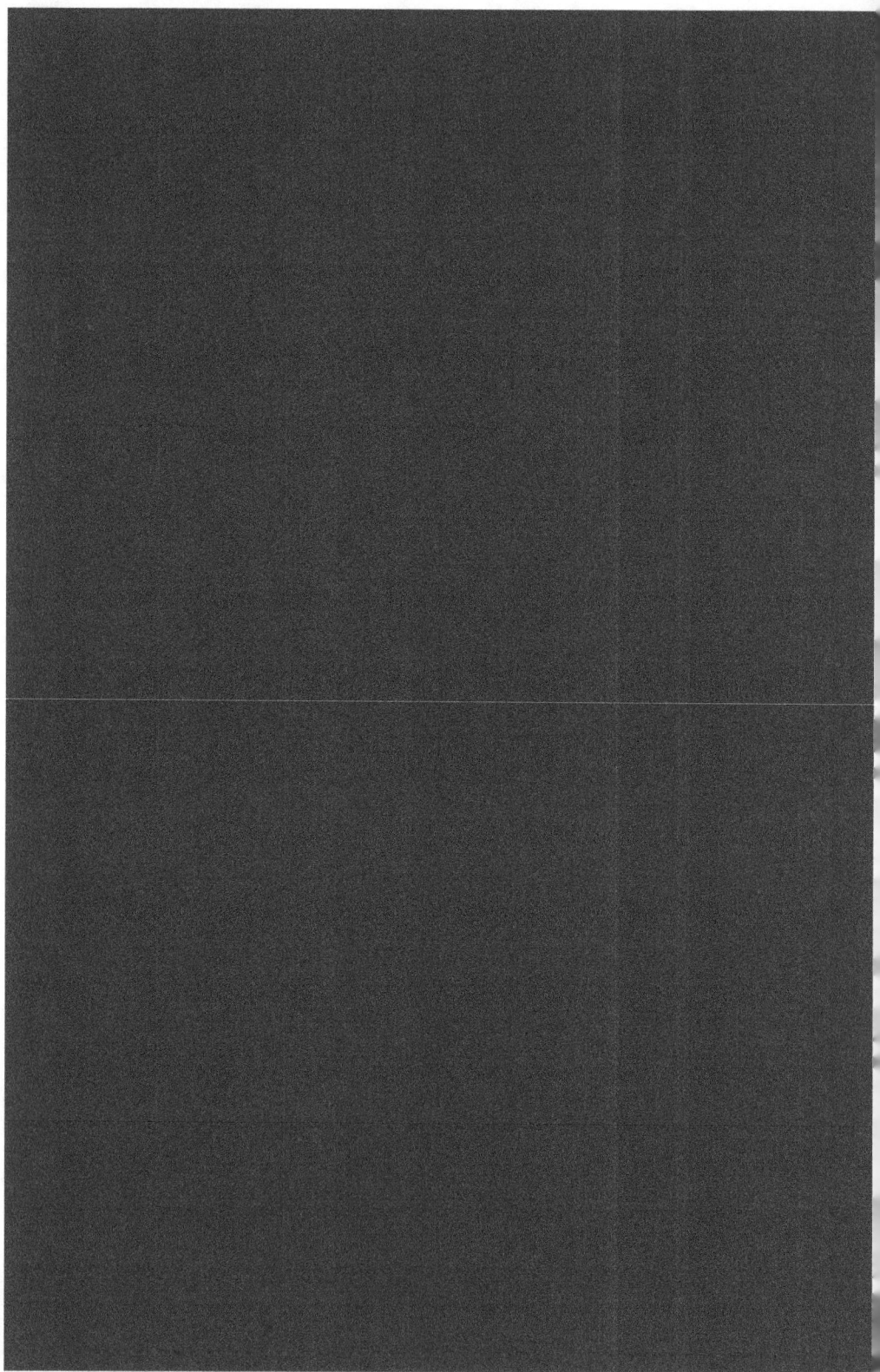

Day 8

DATE _____   S M T W T F S

MORNING THOUGHTS & FEELINGS

_____
_____
_____
_____

MORNING MEAL @ _____

I ATE:
_____
_____

I DRANK:
_____

I FELT:
_____

2-3 HOURS LATER I FELT:
_____

MID MORNING SNACK @ _____

I ATE:
_____
_____

I DRANK:
_____

I FELT:
_____

AFTERNOON MEAL @ _____

I ATE:

_____

_____

I DRANK:

_____

I FELT:

_____

2-3 HOURS LATER I FELT:

_____

AFTERNOON SNACK @ _____

I ATE:

_____

_____

I DRANK:

_____

I FELT:

_____

EVENING MEAL @ _____

I ATE:

_____

_____

_____

I DRANK:

_____

I FELT:

_____

2-3 HOURS LATER I FELT:

_____

HAPPINESS TRACKER - ON A SCALE OF 1-5

Rate the areas below from 1-5, with 1 being least happy & 5 being most happy. Pay close attention to any trends you begin to notice regarding how the things you eat & drink affect the way you feel & your overall happiness.

My morning energy level   ○ ○ ○ ○ ○

My afternoon energy level   ○ ○ ○ ○ ○

My evening energy level   ○ ○ ○ ○ ○

How my body feels   ○ ○ ○ ○ ○

My mental clarity   ○ ○ ○ ○ ○

My emotional stability   ○ ○ ○ ○ ○

My excitement about life   ○ ○ ○ ○ ○

My personal relationships   ○ ○ ○ ○ ○

My professional relationships   ○ ○ ○ ○ ○

My poop   ○ ○ ○ ○ ○

EVENING THOUGHTS & FEELINGS

_____

_____

_____

_____

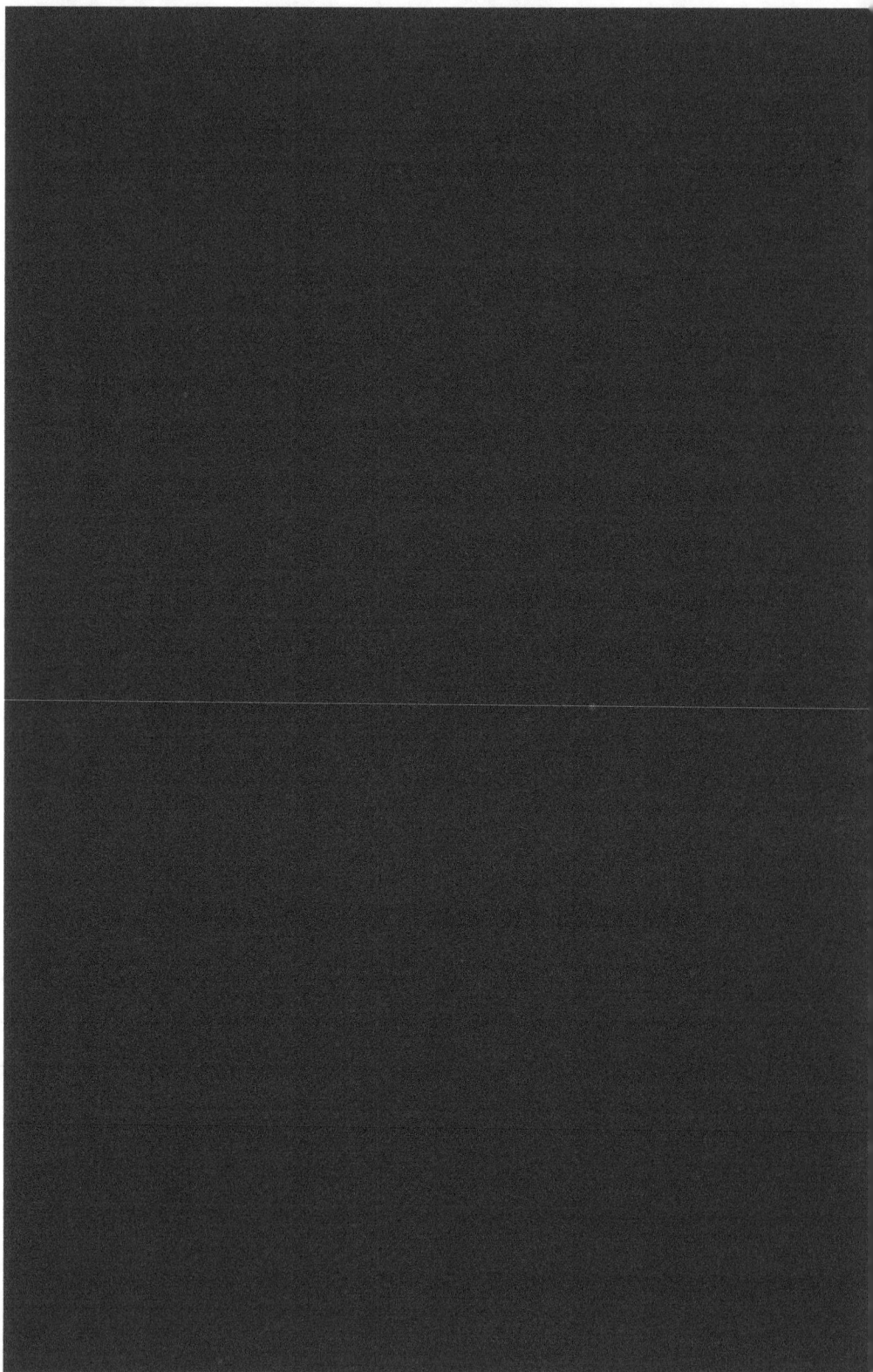

DATE   S M T W T F S

MORNING THOUGHTS & FEELINGS

_____
_____
_____
_____

MORNING MEAL @ _____

I ATE:
_____
_____

I DRANK:
_____

I FELT:
_____

2-3 HOURS LATER I FELT:
_____

MID MORNING SNACK @ _____

I ATE:
_____
_____

I DRANK:
_____

I FELT:
_____

AFTERNOON MEAL @ _____

I ATE:

_____

_____

I DRANK:

_____

I FELT:

_____

2-3 HOURS LATER I FELT:

_____

AFTERNOON SNACK @ _____

I ATE:

_____

_____

I DRANK:

_____

I FELT:

_____

EVENING MEAL @ _____

I ATE:

_____

_____

I DRANK:

_____

I FELT:

_____

2-3 HOURS LATER I FELT:

_____

HAPPINESS TRACKER - ON A SCALE OF 1-5

Rate the areas below from 1-5, with 1 being least happy & 5 being most happy. Pay close attention to any trends you begin to notice regarding how the things you eat & drink affect the way you feel & your overall happiness.

My morning energy level   ○ ○ ○ ○ ○

My afternoon energy level   ○ ○ ○ ○ ○

My evening energy level   ○ ○ ○ ○ ○

How my body feels   ○ ○ ○ ○ ○

My mental clarity   ○ ○ ○ ○ ○

My emotional stability   ○ ○ ○ ○ ○

My excitement about life   ○ ○ ○ ○ ○

My personal relationships   ○ ○ ○ ○ ○

My professional relationships   ○ ○ ○ ○ ○

My poop   ○ ○ ○ ○ ○

EVENING THOUGHTS & FEELINGS

_____

_____

_____

_____

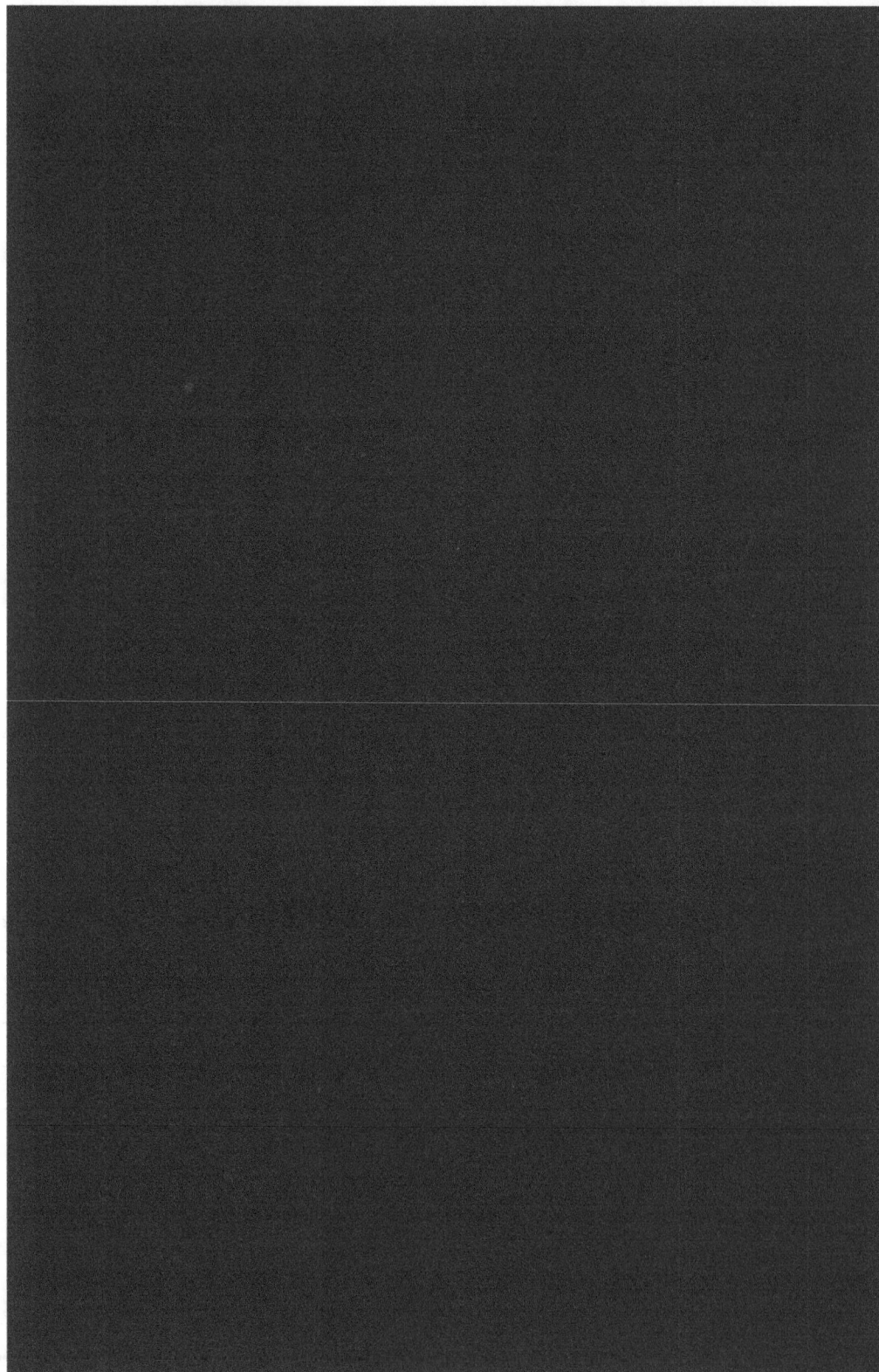

DATE _____   S M T W T F S

MORNING THOUGHTS & FEELINGS

_____
_____
_____
_____

MORNING MEAL @ _____

I ATE:

_____
_____

I DRANK:

_____

I FELT:

_____

2-3 HOURS LATER I FELT:

_____

MID MORNING SNACK @ _____

I ATE:

_____
_____

I DRANK:

_____

I FELT:

_____

AFTERNOON MEAL @ _____

I ATE:

_____
_____

I DRANK:

_____

I FELT:

_____

2-3 HOURS LATER I FELT:

_____

AFTERNOON SNACK @ _____

I ATE:

_____
_____

I DRANK:

_____

I FELT:

_____

EVENING MEAL @ _____

I ATE:

_____
_____

I DRANK:

_____

I FELT:

_____

2-3 HOURS LATER I FELT:

_____

HAPPINESS TRACKER - ON A SCALE OF 1-5

Rate the areas below from 1-5, with 1 being least happy & 5 being most happy. Pay close attention to any trends you begin to notice regarding how the things you eat & drink affect the way you feel & your overall happiness.

My morning energy level ○ ○ ○ ○ ○

My afternoon energy level ○ ○ ○ ○ ○

My evening energy level ○ ○ ○ ○ ○

How my body feels ○ ○ ○ ○ ○

My mental clarity ○ ○ ○ ○ ○

My emotional stability ○ ○ ○ ○ ○

My excitement about life ○ ○ ○ ○ ○

My personal relationships ○ ○ ○ ○ ○

My professional relationships ○ ○ ○ ○ ○

My poop ○ ○ ○ ○ ○

EVENING THOUGHTS & FEELINGS

_____

_____

_____

_____

DATE _____   **S M T W T F S**

MORNING THOUGHTS & FEELINGS

_____
_____
_____
_____

MORNING MEAL @ _____

I ATE:
_____
_____

I DRANK:
_____

I FELT:
_____

2-3 HOURS LATER I FELT:
_____

MID MORNING SNACK @ _____

I ATE:
_____
_____

I DRANK:
_____

I FELT:
_____

AFTERNOON MEAL @ _____

I ATE:

_____
_____

I DRANK:

_____

I FELT:

_____

2-3 HOURS LATER I FELT:

_____

AFTERNOON SNACK @ _____

I ATE:

_____
_____

I DRANK:

_____

I FELT:

_____

EVENING MEAL @ _____

I ATE:

_____
_____

I DRANK:

_____

I FELT:

_____

2-3 HOURS LATER I FELT:

_____

HAPPINESS TRACKER - ON A SCALE OF 1-5

Rate the areas below from 1-5, with 1 being least happy & 5 being most happy. Pay close attention to any trends you begin to notice regarding how the things you eat & drink affect the way you feel & your overall happiness.

My morning energy level	○ ○ ○ ○ ○
My afternoon energy level	○ ○ ○ ○ ○
My evening energy level	○ ○ ○ ○ ○
How my body feels	○ ○ ○ ○ ○
My mental clarity	○ ○ ○ ○ ○
My emotional stability	○ ○ ○ ○ ○
My excitement about life	○ ○ ○ ○ ○
My personal relationships	○ ○ ○ ○ ○
My professional relationships	○ ○ ○ ○ ○
My poop	○ ○ ○ ○ ○

EVENING THOUGHTS & FEELINGS

_____

_____

_____

_____

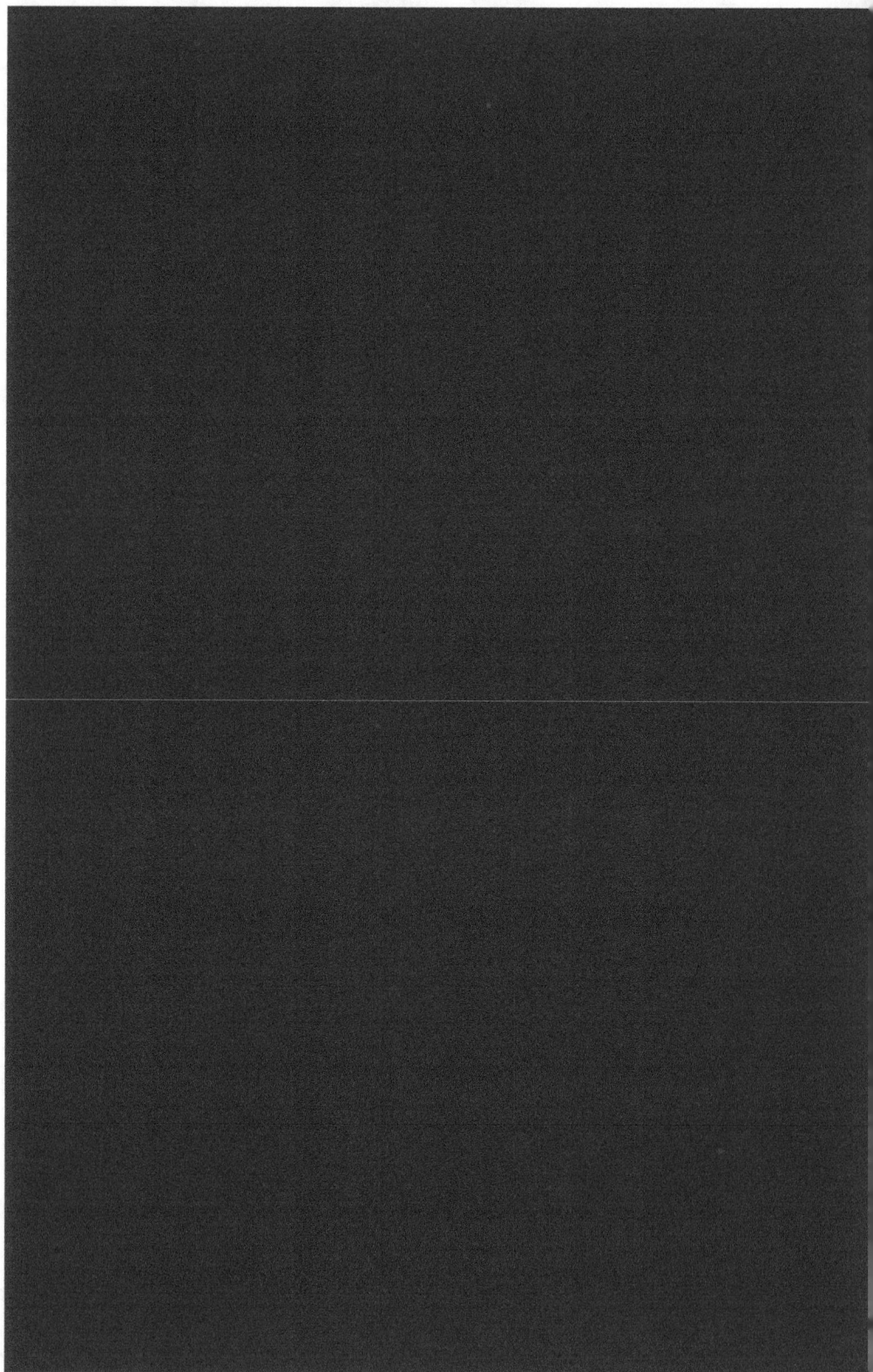

DATE _____   S M T W T F S

MORNING THOUGHTS & FEELINGS

_____

_____

_____

_____

MORNING MEAL @ _____

I ATE:

_____

_____

I DRANK:

_____

I FELT:

_____

2-3 HOURS LATER I FELT:

_____

MID MORNING SNACK @ _____

I ATE:

_____

_____

I DRANK:

_____

I FELT:

_____

AFTERNOON MEAL @ _____

I ATE:

_____

_____

I DRANK:

_____

I FELT:

_____

2-3 HOURS LATER I FELT:

_____

AFTERNOON SNACK @ _____

I ATE:

_____

_____

I DRANK:

_____

I FELT:

_____

EVENING MEAL @ _____

I ATE:

_____

_____

I DRANK:

_____

I FELT:

_____

2-3 HOURS LATER I FELT:

_____

HAPPINESS TRACKER - ON A SCALE OF 1-5

Rate the areas below from 1-5, with 1 being least happy & 5 being most happy. Pay close attention to any trends you begin to notice regarding how the things you eat & drink affect the way you feel & your overall happiness.

My morning energy level	○ ○ ○ ○ ○
My afternoon energy level	○ ○ ○ ○ ○
My evening energy level	○ ○ ○ ○ ○
How my body feels	○ ○ ○ ○ ○
My mental clarity	○ ○ ○ ○ ○
My emotional stability	○ ○ ○ ○ ○
My excitement about life	○ ○ ○ ○ ○
My personal relationships	○ ○ ○ ○ ○
My professional relationships	○ ○ ○ ○ ○
My poop	○ ○ ○ ○ ○

EVENING THOUGHTS & FEELINGS

_____

_____

_____

_____

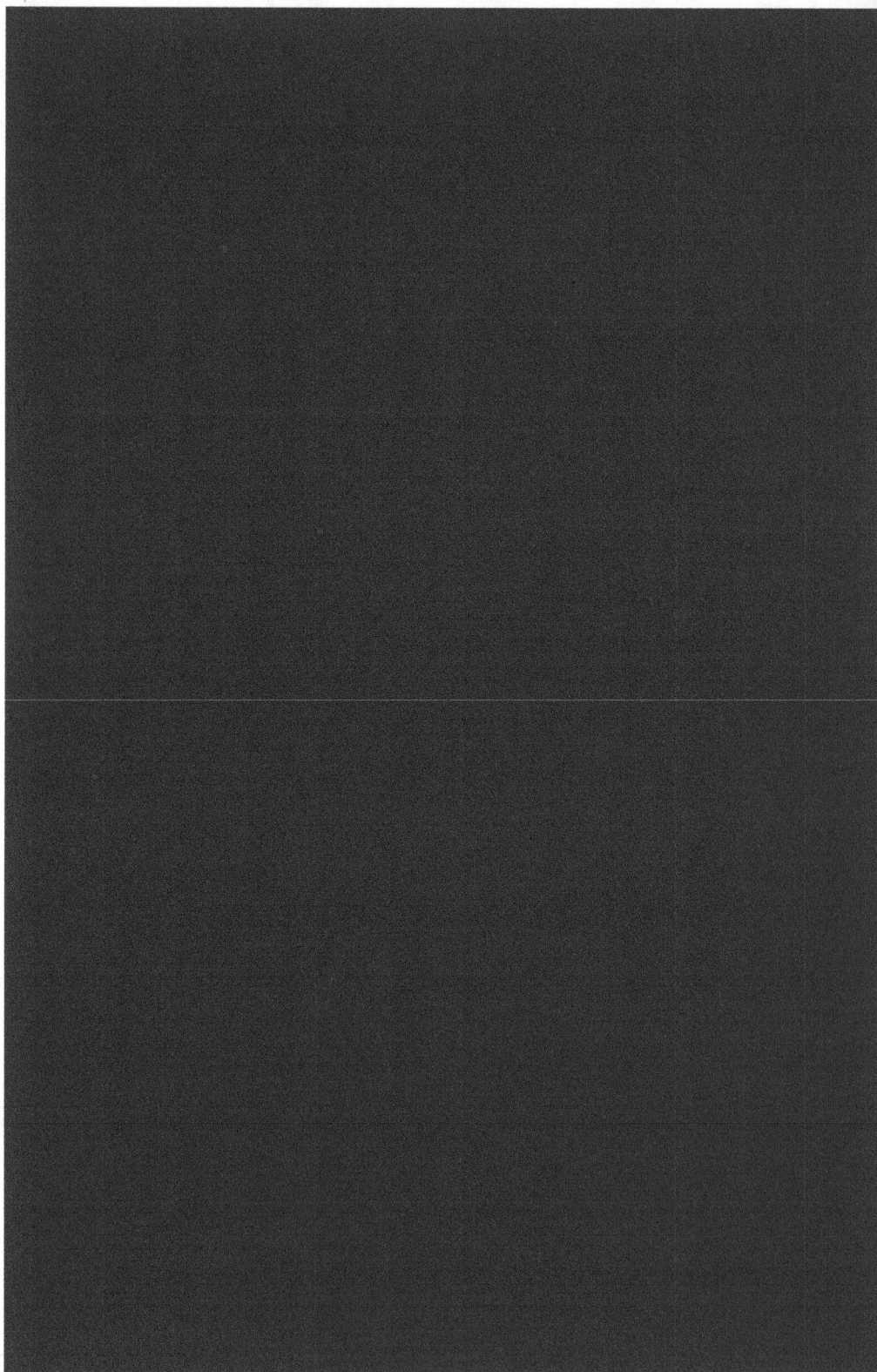

DATE _____   S   M   T   W   T   F   S

MORNING THOUGHTS & FEELINGS

_____
_____
_____
_____

MORNING MEAL @ _____

I ATE:
_____
_____

I DRANK:
_____

I FELT:
_____

2-3 HOURS LATER I FELT:
_____

MID MORNING SNACK @ _____

I ATE:
_____
_____

I DRANK:
_____

I FELT:
_____

AFTERNOON MEAL @ _____

I ATE:

_____

_____

I DRANK:

_____

I FELT:

_____

2-3 HOURS LATER I FELT:

_____

AFTERNOON SNACK @ _____

I ATE:

_____

_____

I DRANK:

_____

I FELT:

_____

EVENING MEAL @ _____

I ATE:

_____

_____

I DRANK:

_____

I FELT:

_____

2-3 HOURS LATER I FELT:

_____

HAPPINESS TRACKER - ON A SCALE OF 1-5

Rate the areas below from 1-5, with 1 being least happy & 5 being most happy. Pay close attention to any trends you begin to notice regarding how the things you eat & drink affect the way you feel & your overall happiness.

My morning energy level   ○ ○ ○ ○ ○

My afternoon energy level   ○ ○ ○ ○ ○

My evening energy level   ○ ○ ○ ○ ○

How my body feels   ○ ○ ○ ○ ○

My mental clarity   ○ ○ ○ ○ ○

My emotional stability   ○ ○ ○ ○ ○

My excitement about life   ○ ○ ○ ○ ○

My personal relationships   ○ ○ ○ ○ ○

My professional relationships   ○ ○ ○ ○ ○

My poop   ○ ○ ○ ○ ○

EVENING THOUGHTS & FEELINGS

_____

_____

_____

_____

DATE _____   **S   M   T   W   T   F   S**

MORNING THOUGHTS & FEELINGS

_____
_____
_____
_____

MORNING MEAL @ _____

I ATE:
_____
_____

I DRANK:
_____

I FELT:
_____

2-3 HOURS LATER I FELT:
_____

MID MORNING SNACK @ _____

I ATE:
_____
_____

I DRANK:
_____

I FELT:
_____

AFTERNOON MEAL @ _____

I ATE:

_____
_____

I DRANK:

_____

I FELT:

_____

2-3 HOURS LATER I FELT:

_____

AFTERNOON SNACK @ _____

I ATE:

_____
_____

I DRANK:

_____

I FELT:

_____

EVENING MEAL @ _____

I ATE:

_____
_____

I DRANK:

_____

I FELT:

_____

2-3 HOURS LATER I FELT:

_____

HAPPINESS TRACKER - ON A SCALE OF 1-5

Rate the areas below from 1-5, with 1 being least happy & 5 being most happy. Pay close attention to any trends you begin to notice regarding how the things you eat & drink affect the way you feel & your overall happiness.

My morning energy level   ◯ ◯ ◯ ◯ ◯

My afternoon energy level   ◯ ◯ ◯ ◯ ◯

My evening energy level   ◯ ◯ ◯ ◯ ◯

How my body feels   ◯ ◯ ◯ ◯ ◯

My mental clarity   ◯ ◯ ◯ ◯ ◯

My emotional stability   ◯ ◯ ◯ ◯ ◯

My excitement about life   ◯ ◯ ◯ ◯ ◯

My personal relationships   ◯ ◯ ◯ ◯ ◯

My professional relationships ◯ ◯ ◯ ◯ ◯

My poop   ◯ ◯ ◯ ◯ ◯

EVENING THOUGHTS & FEELINGS

_____

_____

_____

_____

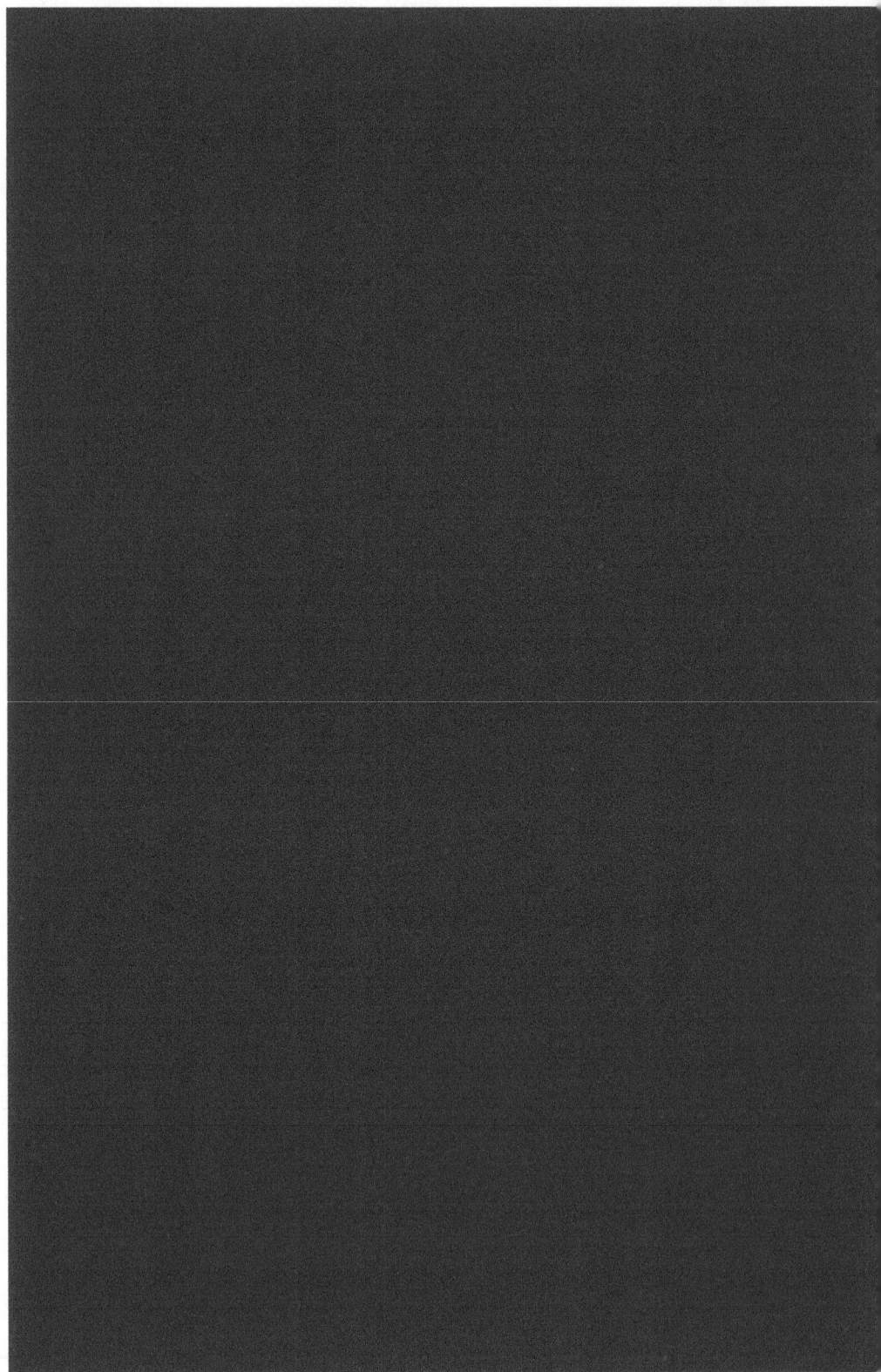

Well done!

You did it!

That's 2 weeks of tracking your thoughts, feelings, emotions, and eating habits.

Have you noticed any trends in what you're eating & how you're feeling?

It's important to recognize & appreciate the amazing progress you're making every single day.

How are you treating yourself?

Whether your idea of self-care is a day hike, a kayak excursion, or taking a good book to the beach - Treat yourself!

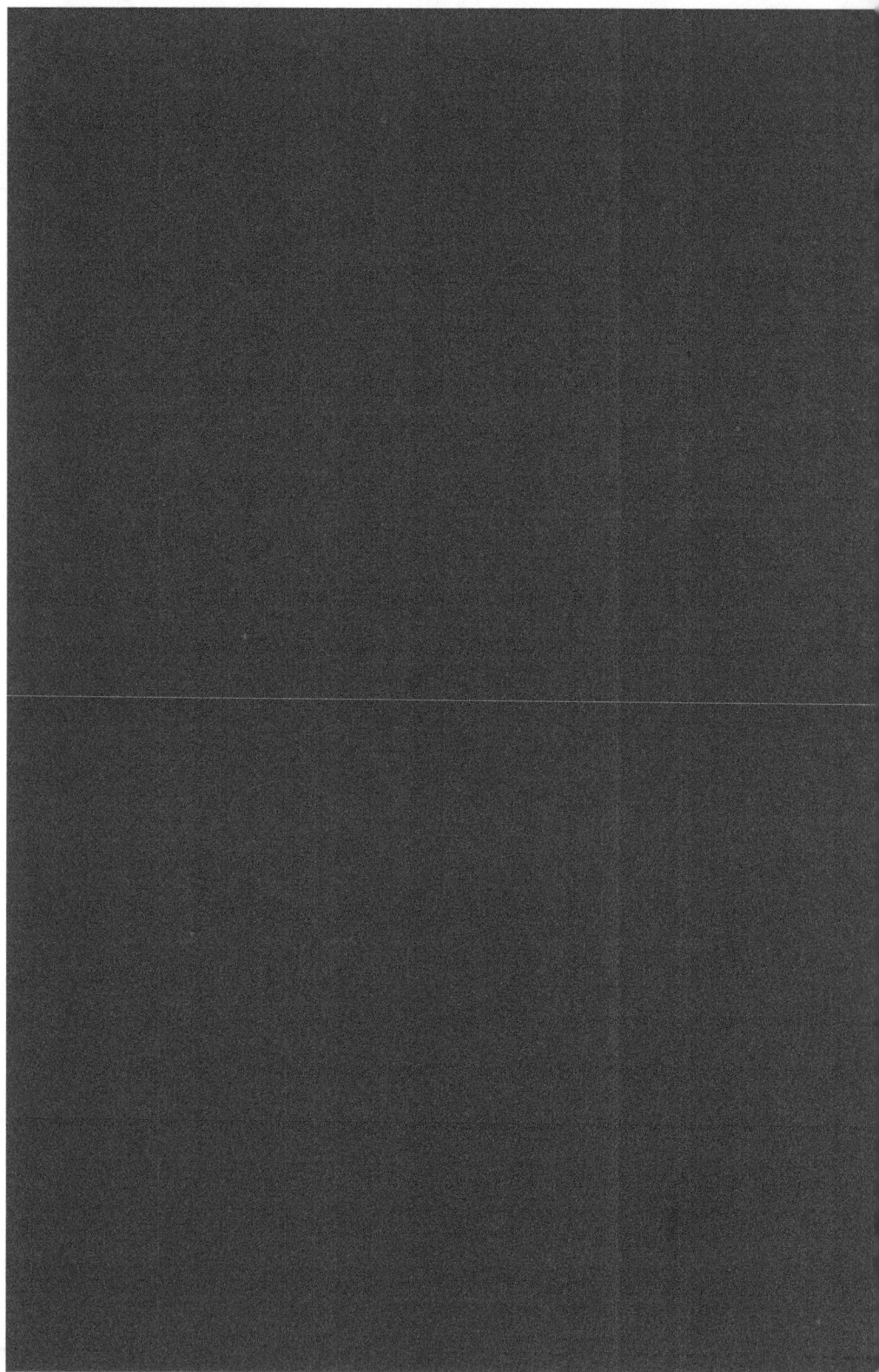

DATE   **S   M   T   W   T   F   S**

MORNING THOUGHTS & FEELINGS

_____

_____

_____

_____

MORNING MEAL @ _____

I ATE:

_____

_____

I DRANK:

_____

I FELT:

_____

2-3 HOURS LATER I FELT:

_____

MID MORNING SNACK @ _____

I ATE:

_____

_____

I DRANK:

_____

I FELT:

_____

AFTERNOON MEAL @ _____

I ATE:

_____

_____

I DRANK:

_____

I FELT:

_____

2-3 HOURS LATER I FELT:

_____

AFTERNOON SNACK @ _____

I ATE:

_____

_____

I DRANK:

_____

I FELT:

_____

EVENING MEAL @ _____

I ATE:

_____

_____

I DRANK:

_____

I FELT:

_____

2-3 HOURS LATER I FELT:

_____

HAPPINESS TRACKER - ON A SCALE OF 1-5

Rate the areas below from 1-5, with 1 being least happy & 5 being most happy. Pay close attention to any trends you begin to notice regarding how the things you eat & drink affect the way you feel & your overall happiness.

My morning energy level   ○ ○ ○ ○ ○

My afternoon energy level   ○ ○ ○ ○ ○

My evening energy level   ○ ○ ○ ○ ○

How my body feels   ○ ○ ○ ○ ○

My mental clarity   ○ ○ ○ ○ ○

My emotional stability   ○ ○ ○ ○ ○

My excitement about life   ○ ○ ○ ○ ○

My personal relationships   ○ ○ ○ ○ ○

My professional relationships   ○ ○ ○ ○ ○

My poop   ○ ○ ○ ○ ○

EVENING THOUGHTS & FEELINGS

_____

_____

_____

_____

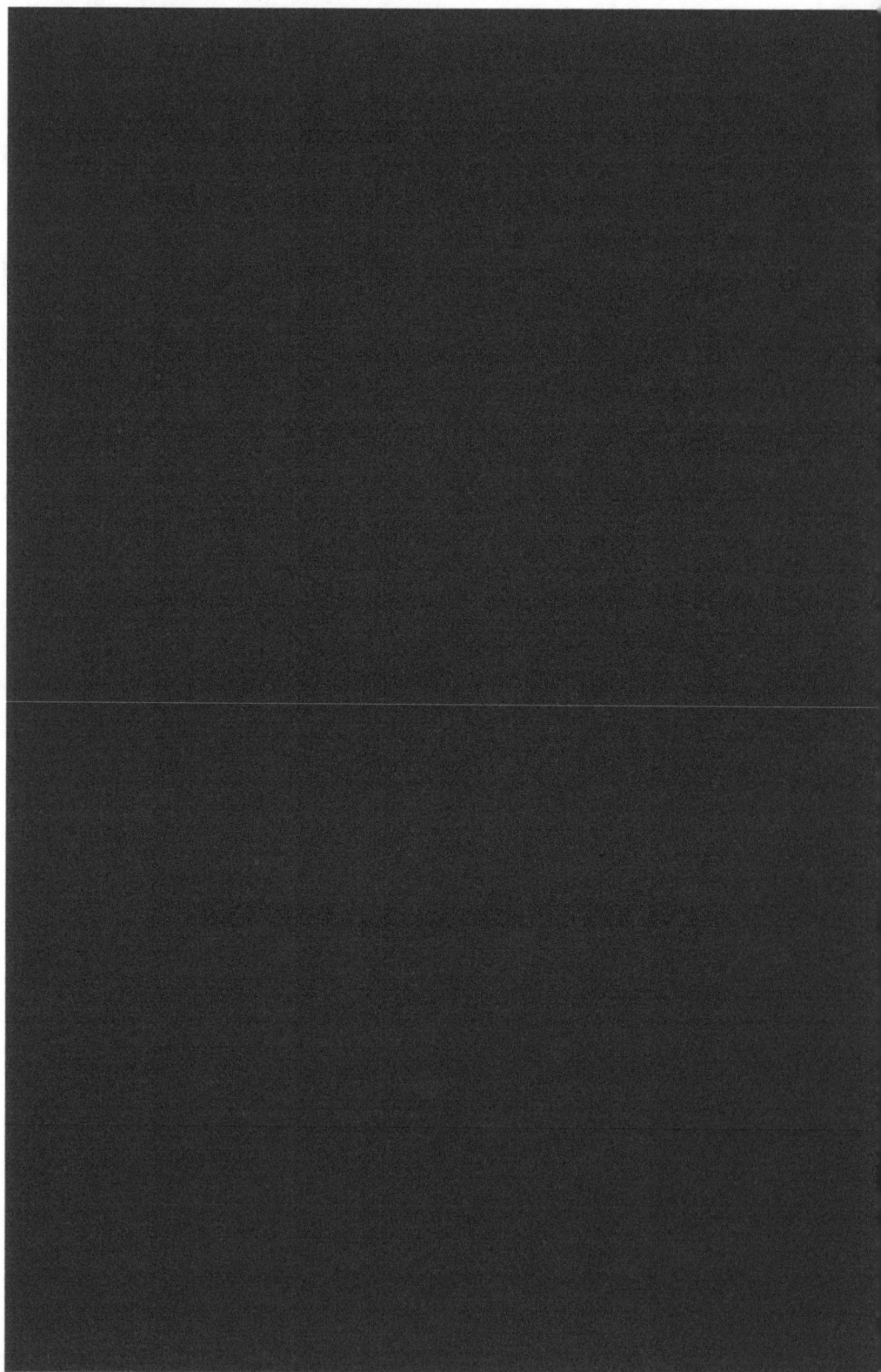

DATE _____   S M T W T F S

MORNING THOUGHTS & FEELINGS

_____

_____

_____

_____

MORNING MEAL @ _____

I ATE:

_____

_____

I DRANK:

_____

I FELT:

_____

2-3 HOURS LATER I FELT:

_____

MID MORNING SNACK @ _____

I ATE:

_____

_____

I DRANK:

_____

I FELT:

_____

AFTERNOON MEAL @ _____

I ATE:

_____
_____

I DRANK:

_____

I FELT:

_____

2-3 HOURS LATER I FELT:

_____

AFTERNOON SNACK @ _____

I ATE:

_____
_____

I DRANK:

_____

I FELT:

_____

EVENING MEAL @ _____

I ATE:

_____
_____

I DRANK:

_____

I FELT:

_____

2-3 HOURS LATER I FELT:

_____

HAPPINESS TRACKER - ON A SCALE OF 1-5

Rate the areas below from 1-5, with 1 being least happy & 5 being most happy. Pay close attention to any trends you begin to notice regarding how the things you eat & drink affect the way you feel & your overall happiness.

My morning energy level	○ ○ ○ ○ ○
My afternoon energy level	○ ○ ○ ○ ○
My evening energy level	○ ○ ○ ○ ○
How my body feels	○ ○ ○ ○ ○
My mental clarity	○ ○ ○ ○ ○
My emotional stability	○ ○ ○ ○ ○
My excitement about life	○ ○ ○ ○ ○
My personal relationships	○ ○ ○ ○ ○
My professional relationships	○ ○ ○ ○ ○
My poop	○ ○ ○ ○ ○

EVENING THOUGHTS & FEELINGS

_____

_____

_____

_____

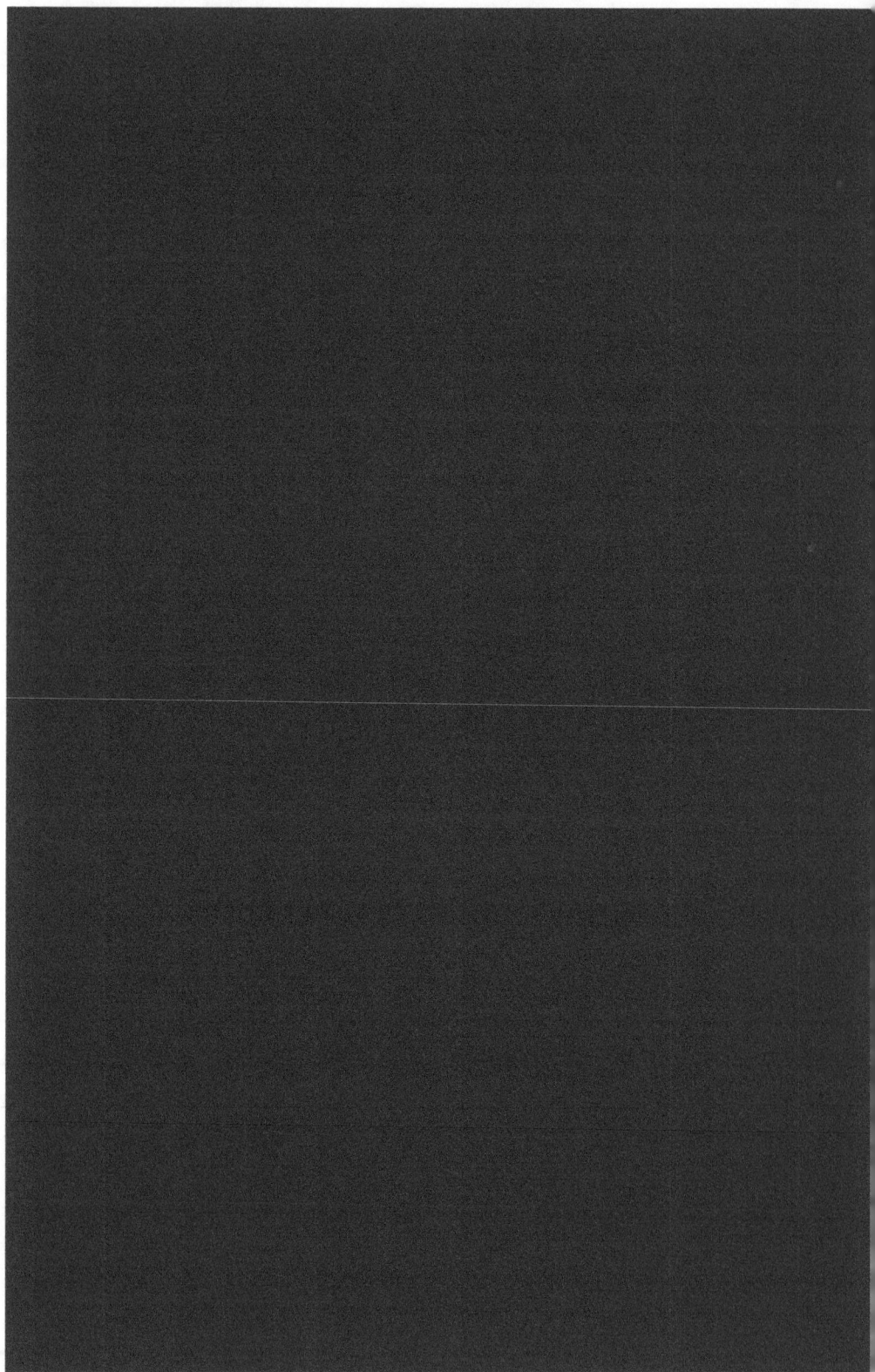

DATE   **S   M   T   W   T   F   S**

MORNING THOUGHTS & FEELINGS

_____
_____
_____
_____

MORNING MEAL @ _____

I ATE:

_____
_____

I DRANK:

_____

I FELT:

_____

2-3 HOURS LATER I FELT:

_____

MID MORNING SNACK @ _____

I ATE:

_____
_____

I DRANK:

_____

I FELT:

_____

AFTERNOON MEAL @ _____

I ATE:

_____
_____

I DRANK:

_____

I FELT:

_____

2-3 HOURS LATER I FELT:

_____

AFTERNOON SNACK @ _____

I ATE:

_____
_____

I DRANK:

_____

I FELT:

_____

EVENING MEAL @ _____

I ATE:

_____
_____

I DRANK:

_____

I FELT:

_____

2-3 HOURS LATER I FELT:

_____

HAPPINESS TRACKER - ON A SCALE OF 1-5

Rate the areas below from 1-5, with 1 being least happy & 5 being most happy. Pay close attention to any trends you begin to notice regarding how the things you eat & drink affect the way you feel & your overall happiness.

My morning energy level   ○ ○ ○ ○ ○

My afternoon energy level   ○ ○ ○ ○ ○

My evening energy level   ○ ○ ○ ○ ○

How my body feels   ○ ○ ○ ○ ○

My mental clarity   ○ ○ ○ ○ ○

My emotional stability   ○ ○ ○ ○ ○

My excitement about life   ○ ○ ○ ○ ○

My personal relationships   ○ ○ ○ ○ ○

My professional relationships   ○ ○ ○ ○ ○

My poop   ○ ○ ○ ○ ○

EVENING THOUGHTS & FEELINGS

_____

_____

_____

_____

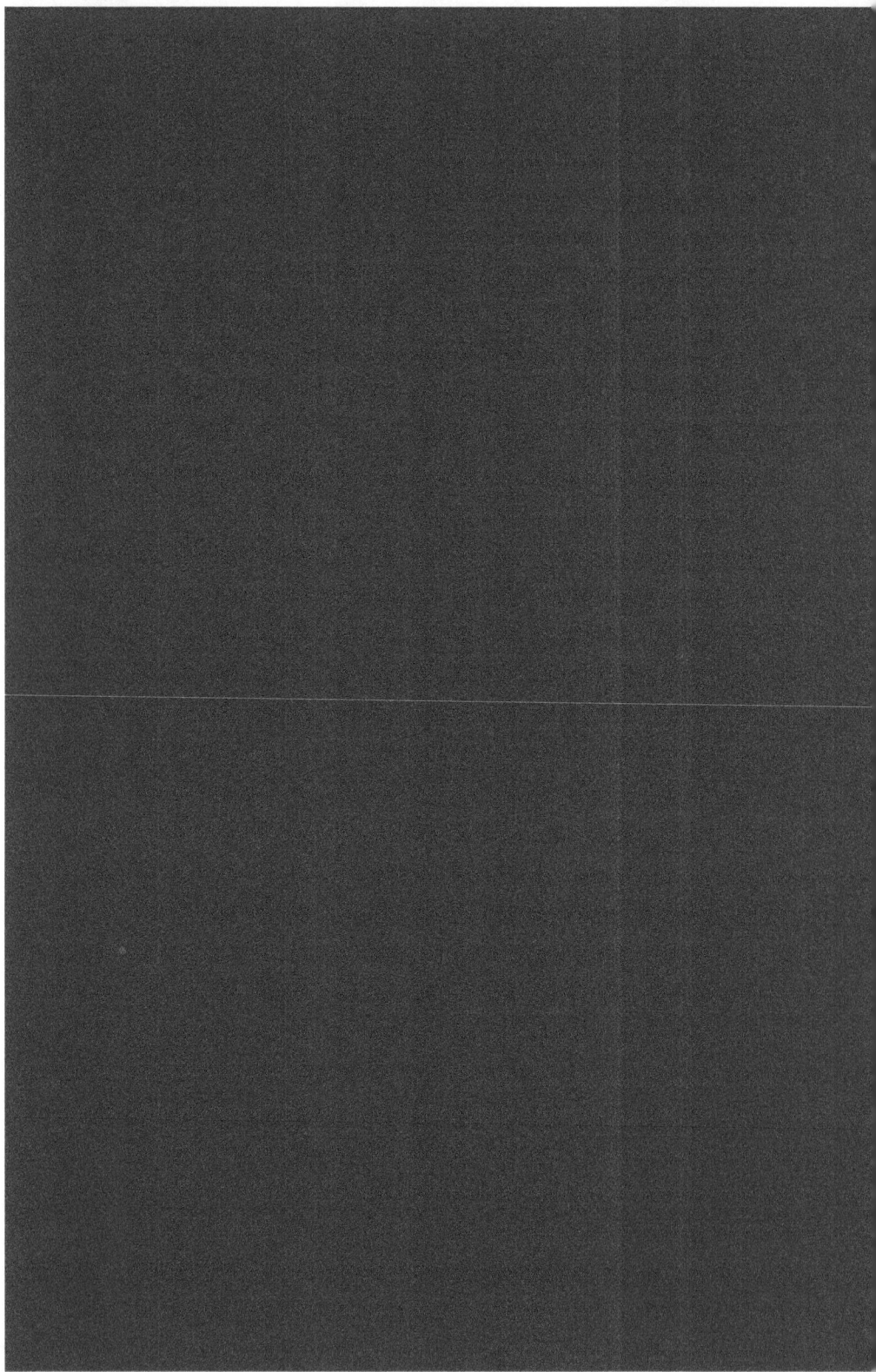

DATE _____   **S M T W T F S**

MORNING THOUGHTS & FEELINGS

_____
_____
_____
_____

MORNING MEAL @ _____

I ATE:
_____
_____

I DRANK:
_____

I FELT:
_____

2-3 HOURS LATER I FELT:
_____

MID MORNING SNACK @ _____

I ATE:
_____
_____

I DRANK:
_____

I FELT:
_____

AFTERNOON MEAL @ _____

I ATE:

_____
_____

I DRANK:

_____

I FELT:

_____

2-3 HOURS LATER I FELT:

_____

AFTERNOON SNACK @ _____

I ATE:

_____
_____

I DRANK:

_____

I FELT:

_____

EVENING MEAL @ _____

I ATE:

_____
_____

I DRANK:

_____

I FELT:

_____

2-3 HOURS LATER I FELT:

_____

HAPPINESS TRACKER - ON A SCALE OF 1-5

Rate the areas below from 1-5, with 1 being least happy & 5 being most happy. Pay close attention to any trends you begin to notice regarding how the things you eat & drink affect the way you feel & your overall happiness.

My morning energy level	○	○	○	○	○
My afternoon energy level	○	○	○	○	○
My evening energy level	○	○	○	○	○
How my body feels	○	○	○	○	○
My mental clarity	○	○	○	○	○
My emotional stability	○	○	○	○	○
My excitement about life	○	○	○	○	○
My personal relationships	○	○	○	○	○
My professional relationships	○	○	○	○	○
My poop	○	○	○	○	○

EVENING THOUGHTS & FEELINGS

_____

_____

_____

_____

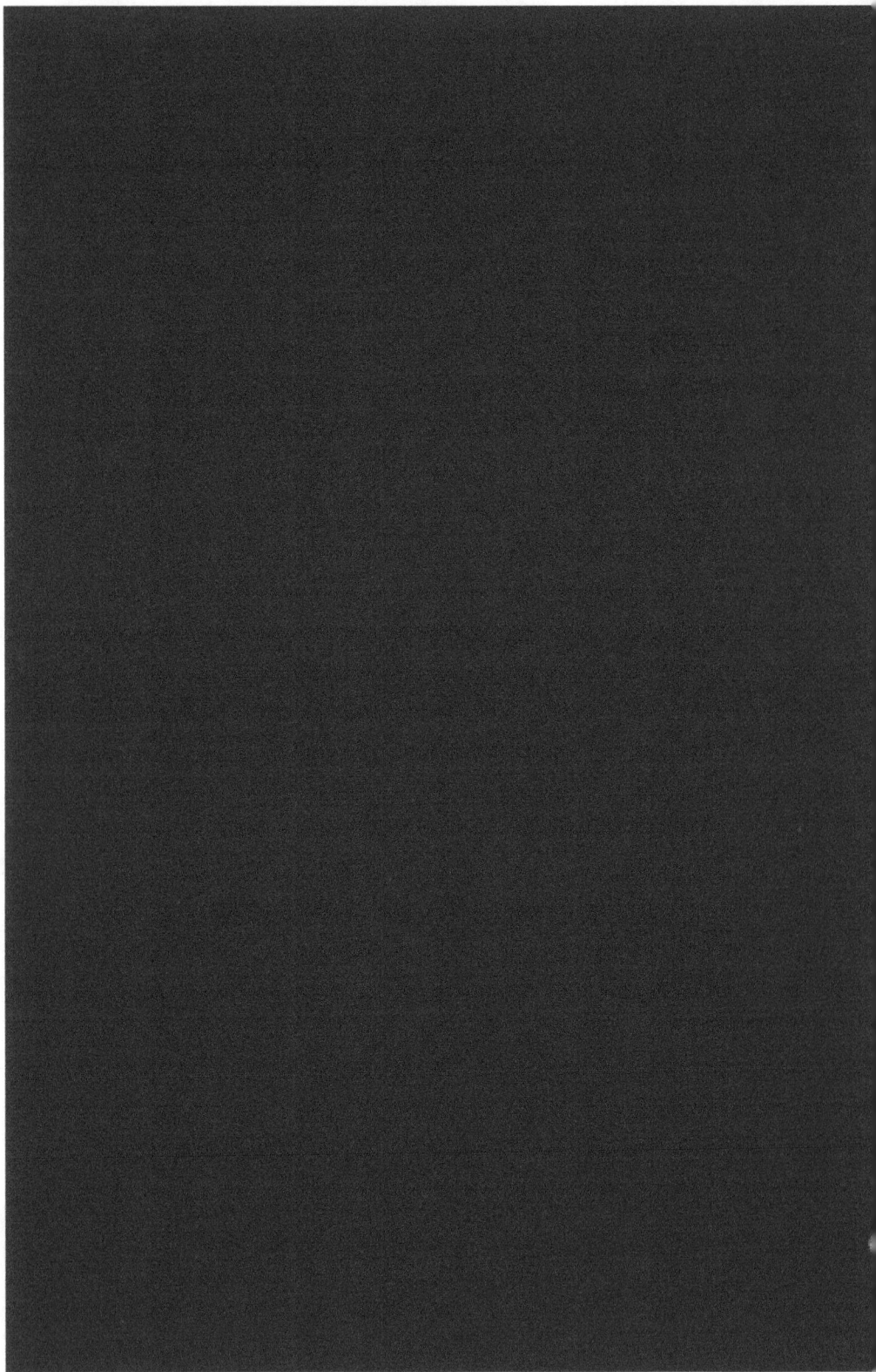

DATE _____   S M T W T F S

MORNING THOUGHTS & FEELINGS

_____
_____
_____
_____

MORNING MEAL @ _____

I ATE:

_____
_____

I DRANK:

_____

I FELT:

_____

2-3 HOURS LATER I FELT:

_____

MID MORNING SNACK @ _____

I ATE:

_____
_____

I DRANK:

_____

I FELT:

_____

AFTERNOON MEAL @ _____

I ATE:

_____

_____

I DRANK:

_____

I FELT:

_____

2-3 HOURS LATER I FELT:

_____

AFTERNOON SNACK @ _____

I ATE:

_____

_____

I DRANK:

_____

I FELT:

_____

EVENING MEAL @ _____

I ATE:

_____

_____

I DRANK:

_____

I FELT:

_____

2-3 HOURS LATER I FELT:

_____

HAPPINESS TRACKER - ON A SCALE OF 1-5

Rate the areas below from 1-5, with 1 being least happy & 5 being most happy. Pay close attention to any trends you begin to notice regarding how the things you eat & drink affect the way you feel & your overall happiness.

My morning energy level   ○ ○ ○ ○ ○

My afternoon energy level   ○ ○ ○ ○ ○

My evening energy level   ○ ○ ○ ○ ○

How my body feels   ○ ○ ○ ○ ○

My mental clarity   ○ ○ ○ ○ ○

My emotional stability   ○ ○ ○ ○ ○

My excitement about life   ○ ○ ○ ○ ○

My personal relationships   ○ ○ ○ ○ ○

My professional relationships   ○ ○ ○ ○ ○

My poop   ○ ○ ○ ○ ○

EVENING THOUGHTS & FEELINGS

_____

_____

_____

_____

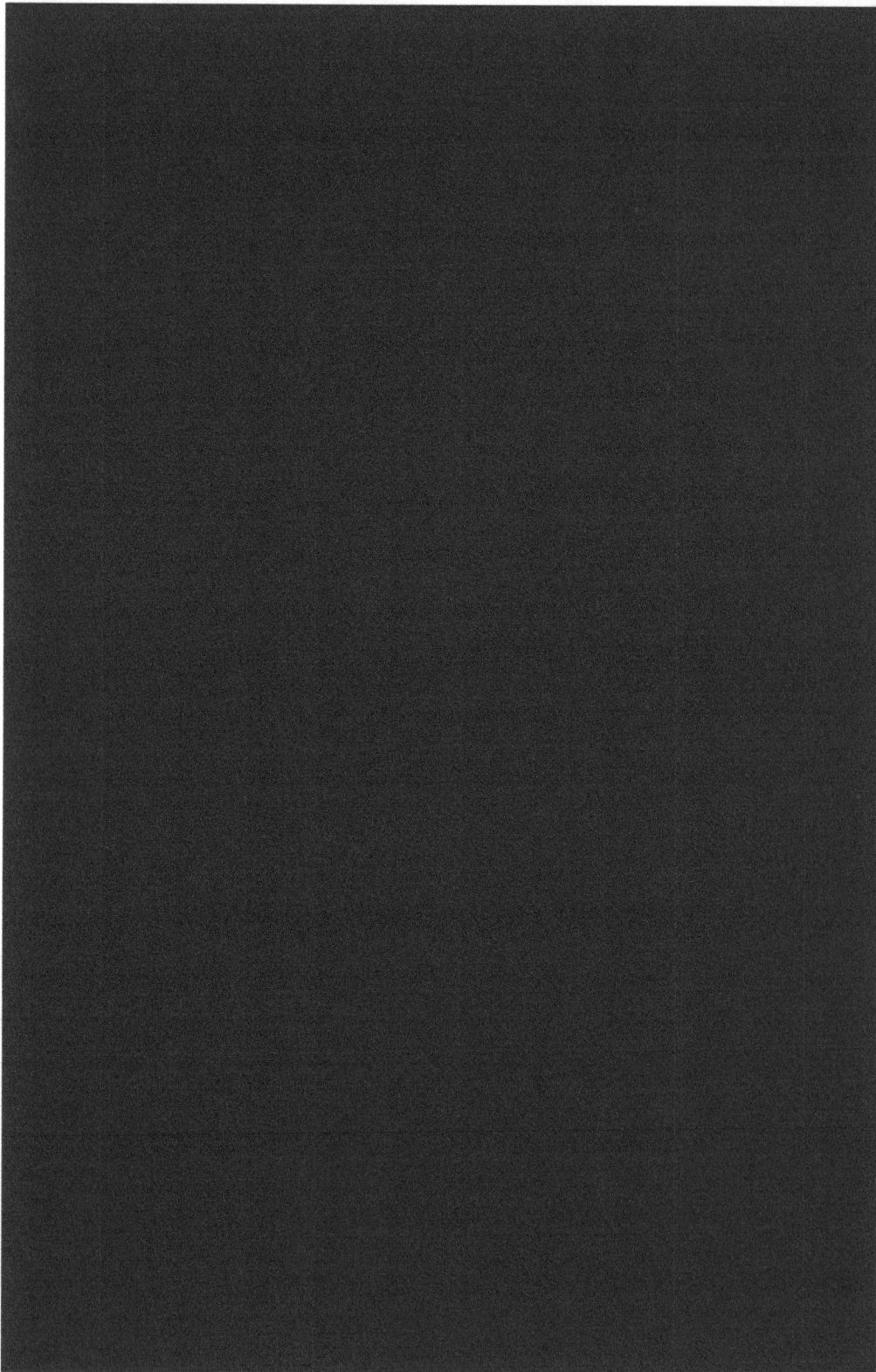

DATE _____ S M T W T F S

MORNING THOUGHTS & FEELINGS

_____
_____
_____
_____

MORNING MEAL @ _____

I ATE:

_____
_____

I DRANK:

_____

I FELT:

_____

2-3 HOURS LATER I FELT:

_____

MID MORNING SNACK @ _____

I ATE:

_____
_____

I DRANK:

_____

I FELT:

_____

AFTERNOON MEAL @ _____

I ATE:

_____

_____

I DRANK:

_____

I FELT:

_____

2-3 HOURS LATER I FELT:

_____

AFTERNOON SNACK @ _____

I ATE:

_____

_____

I DRANK:

_____

I FELT:

_____

EVENING MEAL @ _____

I ATE:

_____

_____

I DRANK:

_____

I FELT:

_____

2-3 HOURS LATER I FELT:

_____

HAPPINESS TRACKER - ON A SCALE OF 1-5

Rate the areas below from 1-5, with 1 being least happy & 5 being most happy. Pay close attention to any trends you begin to notice regarding how the things you eat & drink affect the way you feel & your overall happiness.

My morning energy level   ○ ○ ○ ○ ○

My afternoon energy level   ○ ○ ○ ○ ○

My evening energy level   ○ ○ ○ ○ ○

How my body feels   ○ ○ ○ ○ ○

My mental clarity   ○ ○ ○ ○ ○

My emotional stability   ○ ○ ○ ○ ○

My excitement about life   ○ ○ ○ ○ ○

My personal relationships   ○ ○ ○ ○ ○

My professional relationships   ○ ○ ○ ○ ○

My poop   ○ ○ ○ ○ ○

EVENING THOUGHTS & FEELINGS

_____

_____

_____

_____

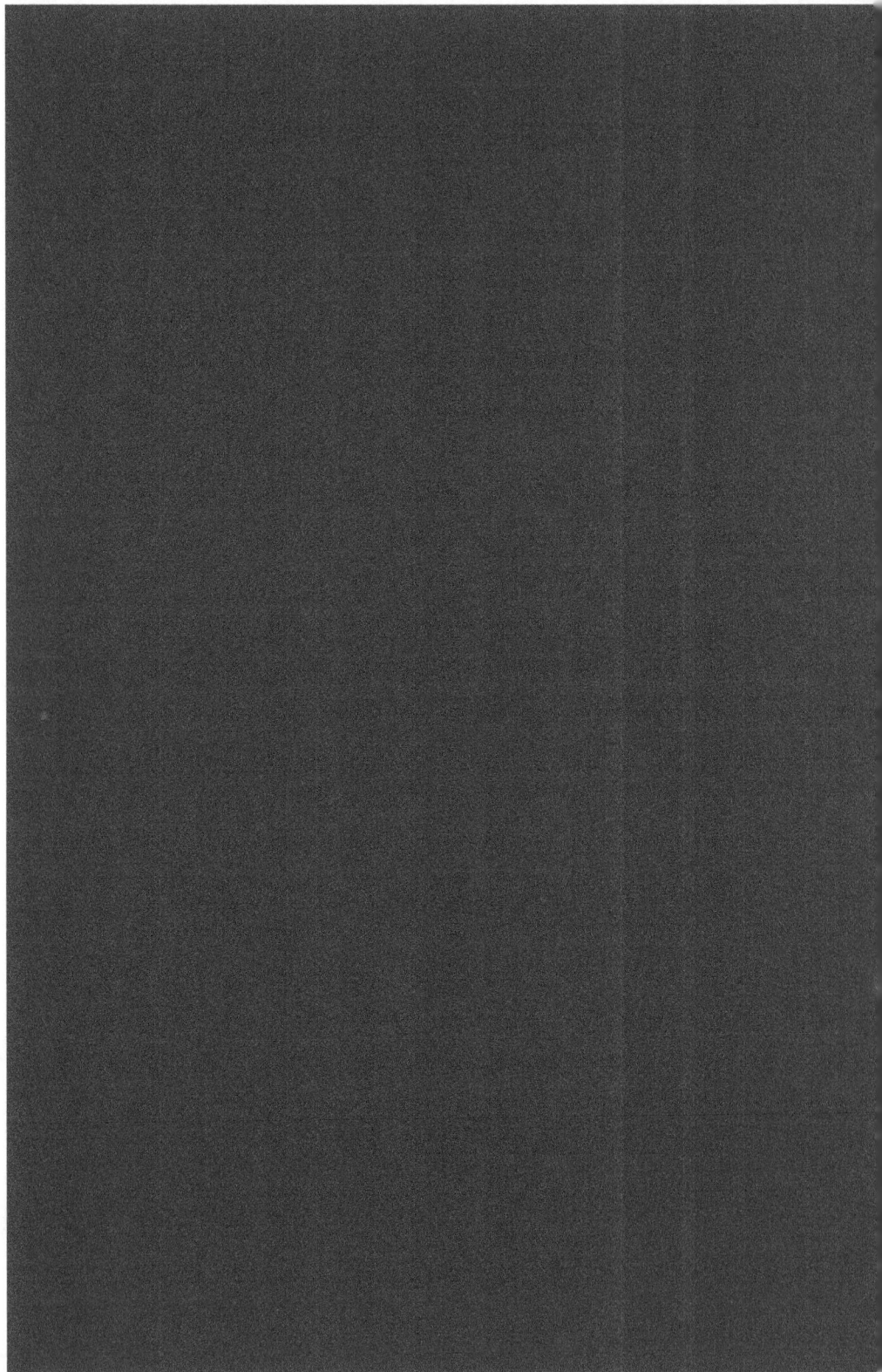

Day 21

DATE   S   M   T   W   T   F   S

MORNING THOUGHTS & FEELINGS

_____
_____
_____
_____

MORNING MEAL @ _____

I ATE:
_____
_____

I DRANK:
_____

I FELT:
_____

2-3 HOURS LATER I FELT:
_____

MID MORNING SNACK @ _____

I ATE:
_____
_____

I DRANK:
_____

I FELT:
_____

AFTERNOON MEAL @ _____

I ATE:

_____
_____

I DRANK:

_____

I FELT:

_____

2-3 HOURS LATER I FELT:

_____

AFTERNOON SNACK @ _____

I ATE:

_____
_____

I DRANK:

_____

I FELT:

_____

EVENING MEAL @ _____

I ATE:

_____
_____

I DRANK:

_____

I FELT:

_____

2-3 HOURS LATER I FELT:

_____

HAPPINESS TRACKER - ON A SCALE OF 1-5

Rate the areas below from 1-5, with 1 being least happy & 5 being most happy. Pay close attention to any trends you begin to notice regarding how the things you eat & drink affect the way you feel & your overall happiness.

My morning energy level	○ ○ ○ ○ ○	
My afternoon energy level	○ ○ ○ ○ ○	
My evening energy level	○ ○ ○ ○ ○	
How my body feels	○ ○ ○ ○ ○	
My mental clarity	○ ○ ○ ○ ○	
My emotional stability	○ ○ ○ ○ ○	
My excitement about life	○ ○ ○ ○ ○	
My personal relationships	○ ○ ○ ○ ○	
My professional relationships	○ ○ ○ ○ ○	
My poop	○ ○ ○ ○ ○	

EVENING THOUGHTS & FEELINGS

_____

_____

_____

_____

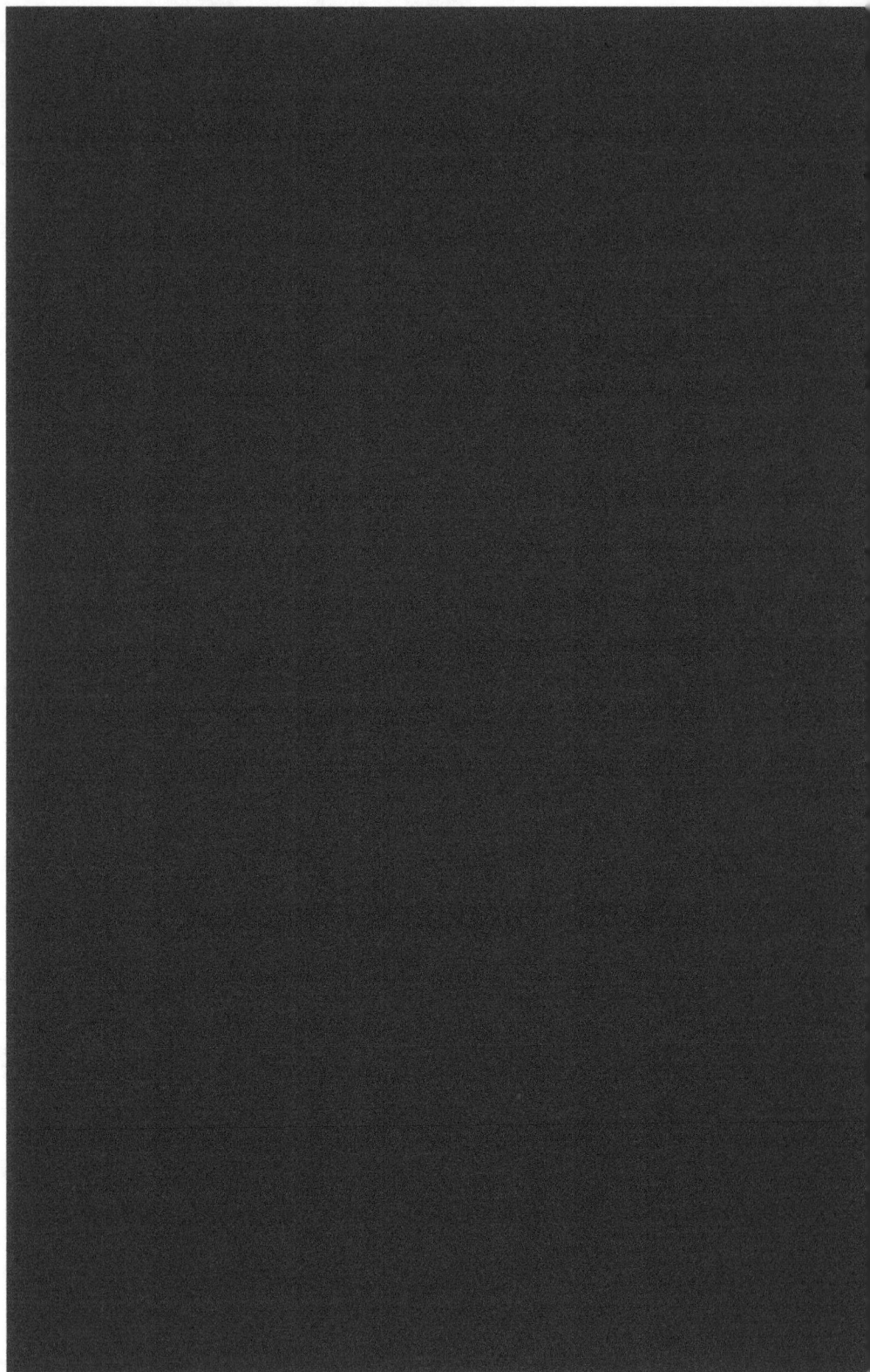

Well done!

You did it!

That's 3 weeks of tracking your happiness & eating habits.

What foods are you finding that leave you feeling energized & fulfilled?

What foods have you noticed leave you feeling not so spectacular?

How are you treating yourself?

Whether your idea of self-care is a mudmask facial, a day of Netflix binging, or taking the dog for a walk in the woods - Treat yourself!

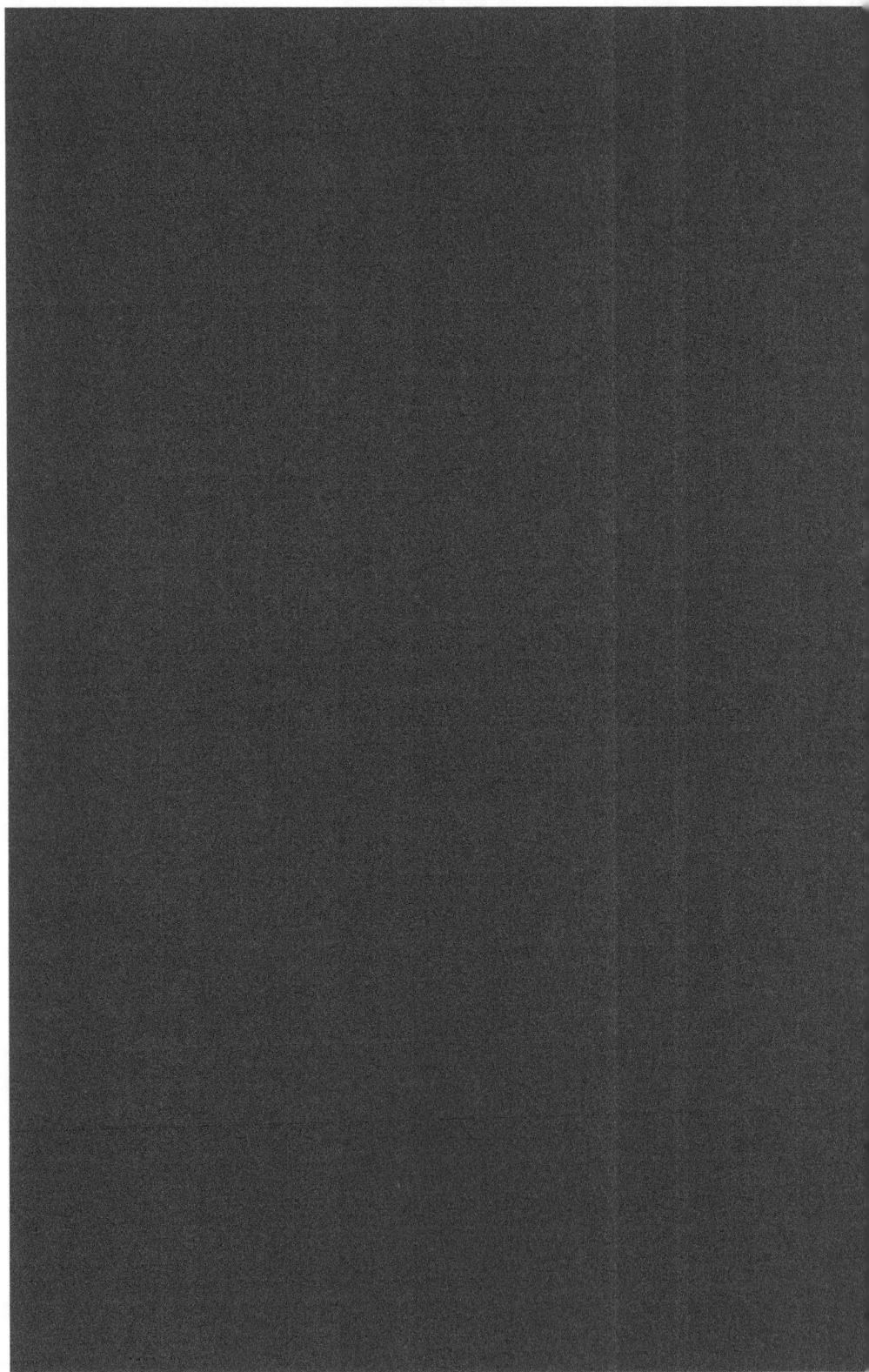

DATE _____   **S   M   T   W   T   F   S**

MORNING THOUGHTS & FEELINGS

_____
_____
_____
_____

MORNING MEAL @ _____

I ATE:

_____
_____

I DRANK:

_____

I FELT:

_____

2-3 HOURS LATER I FELT:

_____

MID MORNING SNACK @ _____

I ATE:

_____
_____

I DRANK:

_____

I FELT:

_____

AFTERNOON MEAL @ _____

I ATE:

_____
_____

I DRANK:

_____

I FELT:

_____

2-3 HOURS LATER I FELT:

_____

AFTERNOON SNACK @ _____

I ATE:

_____
_____

I DRANK:

_____

I FELT:

_____

EVENING MEAL @ _____

I ATE:

_____
_____

I DRANK:

_____

I FELT:

_____

2-3 HOURS LATER I FELT:

_____

HAPPINESS TRACKER - ON A SCALE OF 1-5

Rate the areas below from 1-5, with 1 being least happy & 5 being most happy. Pay close attention to any trends you begin to notice regarding how the things you eat & drink affect the way you feel & your overall happiness.

My morning energy level   ○ ○ ○ ○ ○

My afternoon energy level   ○ ○ ○ ○ ○

My evening energy level   ○ ○ ○ ○ ○

How my body feels   ○ ○ ○ ○ ○

My mental clarity   ○ ○ ○ ○ ○

My emotional stability   ○ ○ ○ ○ ○

My excitement about life   ○ ○ ○ ○ ○

My personal relationships   ○ ○ ○ ○ ○

My professional relationships   ○ ○ ○ ○ ○

My poop   ○ ○ ○ ○ ○

EVENING THOUGHTS & FEELINGS

_____

_____

_____

_____

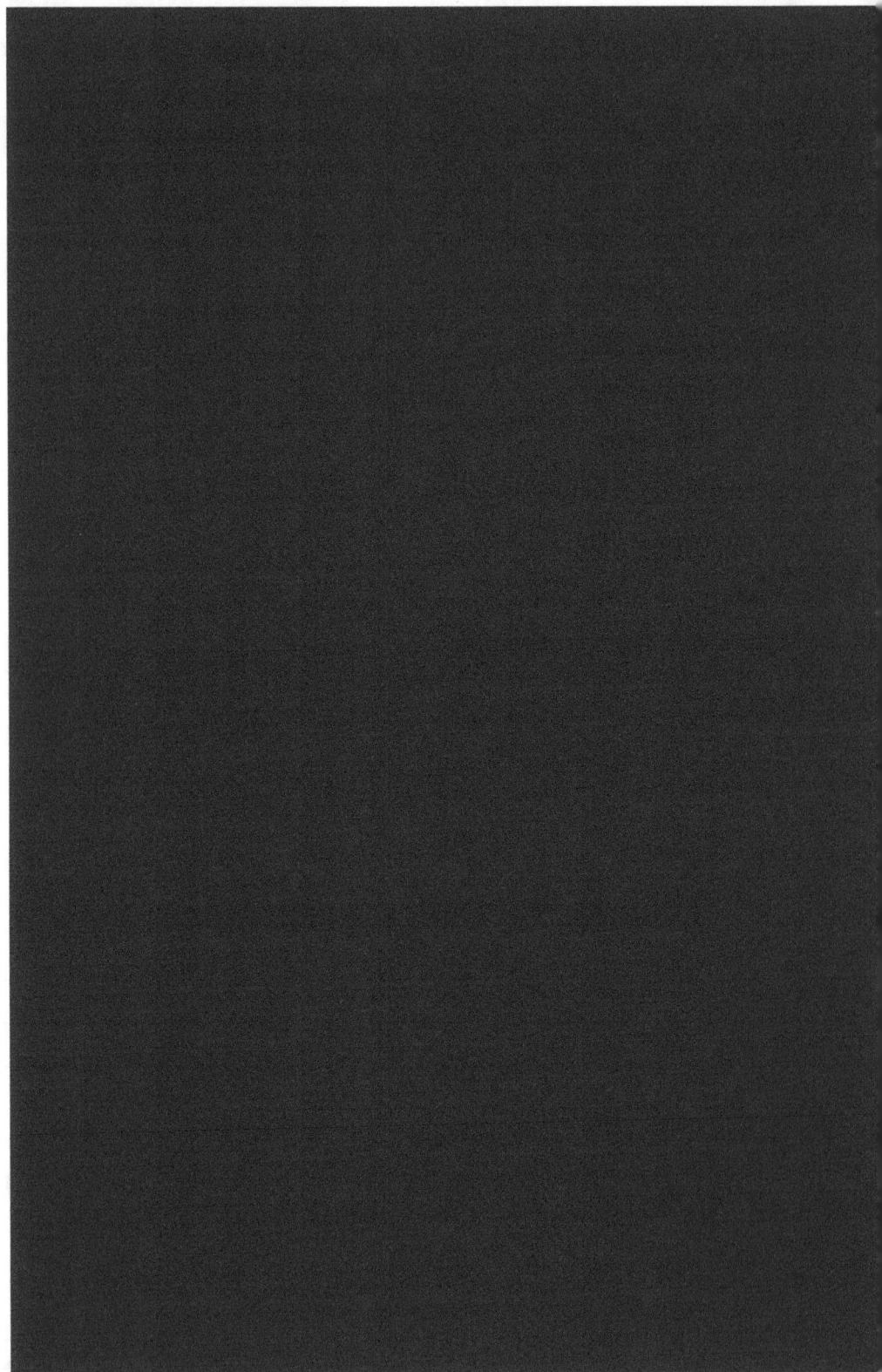

Day 23

DATE   S   M   T   W   T   F   S

MORNING THOUGHTS & FEELINGS

_____

_____

_____

_____

MORNING MEAL @ _____

I ATE:

_____

_____

I DRANK:

_____

I FELT:

_____

2-3 HOURS LATER I FELT:

_____

MID MORNING SNACK @ _____

I ATE:

_____

_____

I DRANK:

_____

I FELT:

_____

AFTERNOON MEAL @ _____

I ATE:

_____
_____

I DRANK:

_____

I FELT:

_____

2-3 HOURS LATER I FELT:

_____

AFTERNOON SNACK @ _____

I ATE:

_____
_____

I DRANK:

_____

I FELT:

_____

EVENING MEAL @ _____

I ATE:

_____
_____

I DRANK:

_____

I FELT:

_____

2-3 HOURS LATER I FELT:

_____

HAPPINESS TRACKER - ON A SCALE OF 1-5

Rate the areas below from 1-5, with 1 being least happy & 5 being most happy. Pay close attention to any trends you begin to notice regarding how the things you eat & drink affect the way you feel & your overall happiness.

My morning energy level ○ ○ ○ ○ ○

My afternoon energy level ○ ○ ○ ○ ○

My evening energy level ○ ○ ○ ○ ○

How my body feels ○ ○ ○ ○ ○

My mental clarity ○ ○ ○ ○ ○

My emotional stability ○ ○ ○ ○ ○

My excitement about life ○ ○ ○ ○ ○

My personal relationships ○ ○ ○ ○ ○

My professional relationships ○ ○ ○ ○ ○

My poop ○ ○ ○ ○ ○

EVENING THOUGHTS & FEELINGS

_____

_____

_____

_____

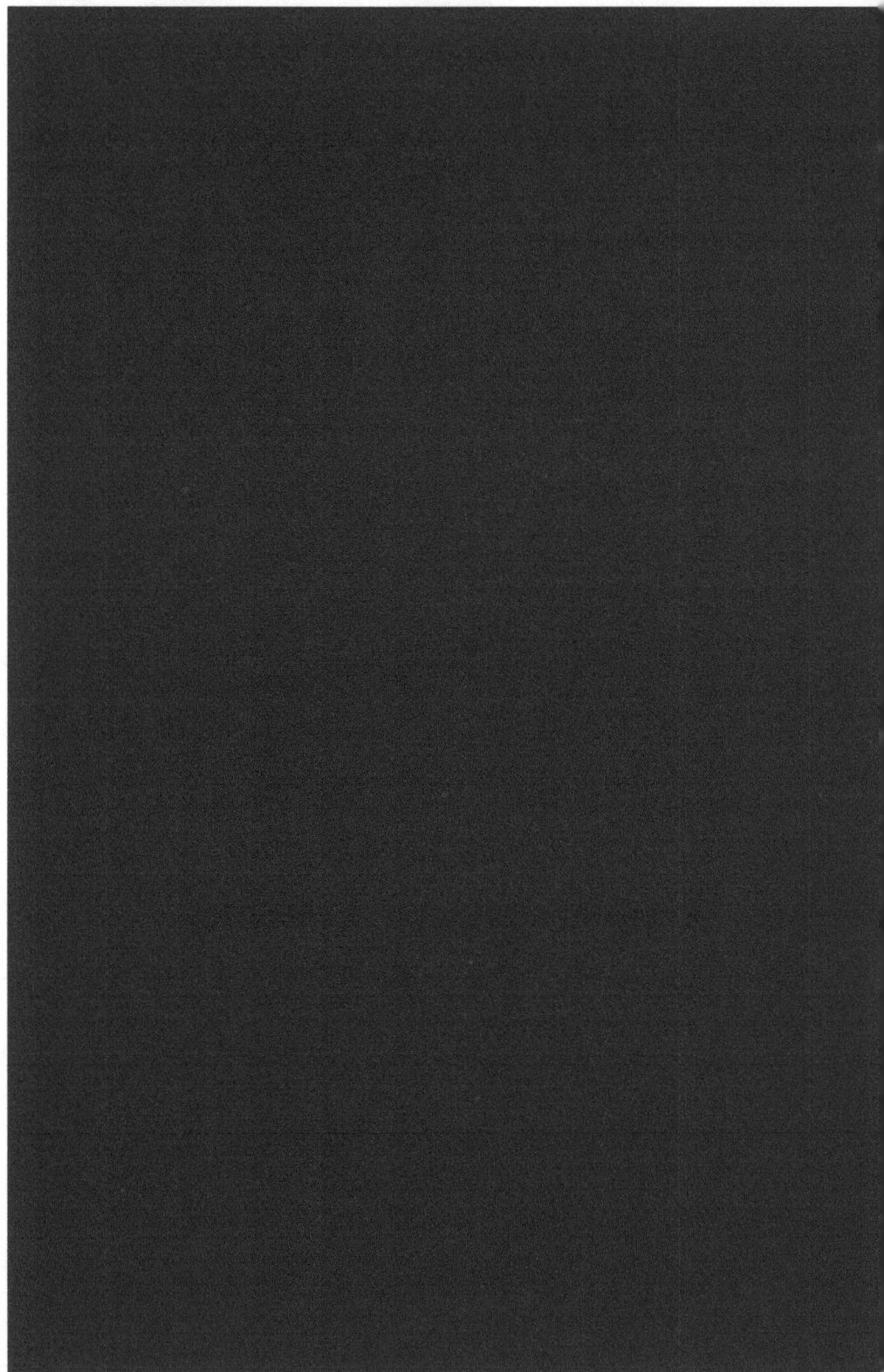

Day 24

DATE _____   **S M T W T F S**

MORNING THOUGHTS & FEELINGS

_____
_____
_____
_____
_____

MORNING MEAL @ _____

I ATE:
_____
_____

I DRANK:
_____

I FELT:
_____

2-3 HOURS LATER I FELT:
_____

MID MORNING SNACK @ _____

I ATE:
_____
_____

I DRANK:
_____

I FELT:
_____

AFTERNOON MEAL @ _____

I ATE:

_____
_____

I DRANK:

_____

I FELT:

_____

2-3 HOURS LATER I FELT:

_____

AFTERNOON SNACK @ _____

I ATE:

_____
_____

I DRANK:

_____

I FELT:

_____

EVENING MEAL @ _____

I ATE:

_____
_____

I DRANK:

_____

I FELT:

_____

2-3 HOURS LATER I FELT:

_____

HAPPINESS TRACKER - ON A SCALE OF 1-5

Rate the areas below from 1-5, with 1 being least happy & 5 being most happy. Pay close attention to any trends you begin to notice regarding how the things you eat & drink affect the way you feel & your overall happiness.

My morning energy level	○	○	○	○	○
My afternoon energy level	○	○	○	○	○
My evening energy level	○	○	○	○	○
How my body feels	○	○	○	○	○
My mental clarity	○	○	○	○	○
My emotional stability	○	○	○	○	○
My excitement about life	○	○	○	○	○
My personal relationships	○	○	○	○	○
My professional relationships	○	○	○	○	○
My poop	○	○	○	○	○

EVENING THOUGHTS & FEELINGS

_____

_____

_____

_____

DATE _____ S M T W T F S

MORNING THOUGHTS & FEELINGS

_____
_____
_____
_____
_____

MORNING MEAL @ _____

I ATE:
_____
_____

I DRANK:
_____

I FELT:
_____

2-3 HOURS LATER I FELT:
_____

MID MORNING SNACK @ _____

I ATE:
_____
_____

I DRANK:
_____

I FELT:
_____

AFTERNOON MEAL @ _____

I ATE:

_____

_____

I DRANK:

_____

I FELT:

_____

2-3 HOURS LATER I FELT:

_____

AFTERNOON SNACK @ _____

I ATE:

_____

_____

I DRANK:

_____

I FELT:

_____

EVENING MEAL @ _____

I ATE:

_____

_____

I DRANK:

_____

I FELT:

_____

2-3 HOURS LATER I FELT:

_____

HAPPINESS TRACKER - ON A SCALE OF 1-5

Rate the areas below from 1-5, with 1 being least happy & 5 being most happy. Pay close attention to any trends you begin to notice regarding how the things you eat & drink affect the way you feel & your overall happiness.

My morning energy level ○ ○ ○ ○ ○

My afternoon energy level ○ ○ ○ ○ ○

My evening energy level ○ ○ ○ ○ ○

How my body feels ○ ○ ○ ○ ○

My mental clarity ○ ○ ○ ○ ○

My emotional stability ○ ○ ○ ○ ○

My excitement about life ○ ○ ○ ○ ○

My personal relationships ○ ○ ○ ○ ○

My professional relationships ○ ○ ○ ○ ○

My poop ○ ○ ○ ○ ○

EVENING THOUGHTS & FEELINGS

_____

_____

_____

_____

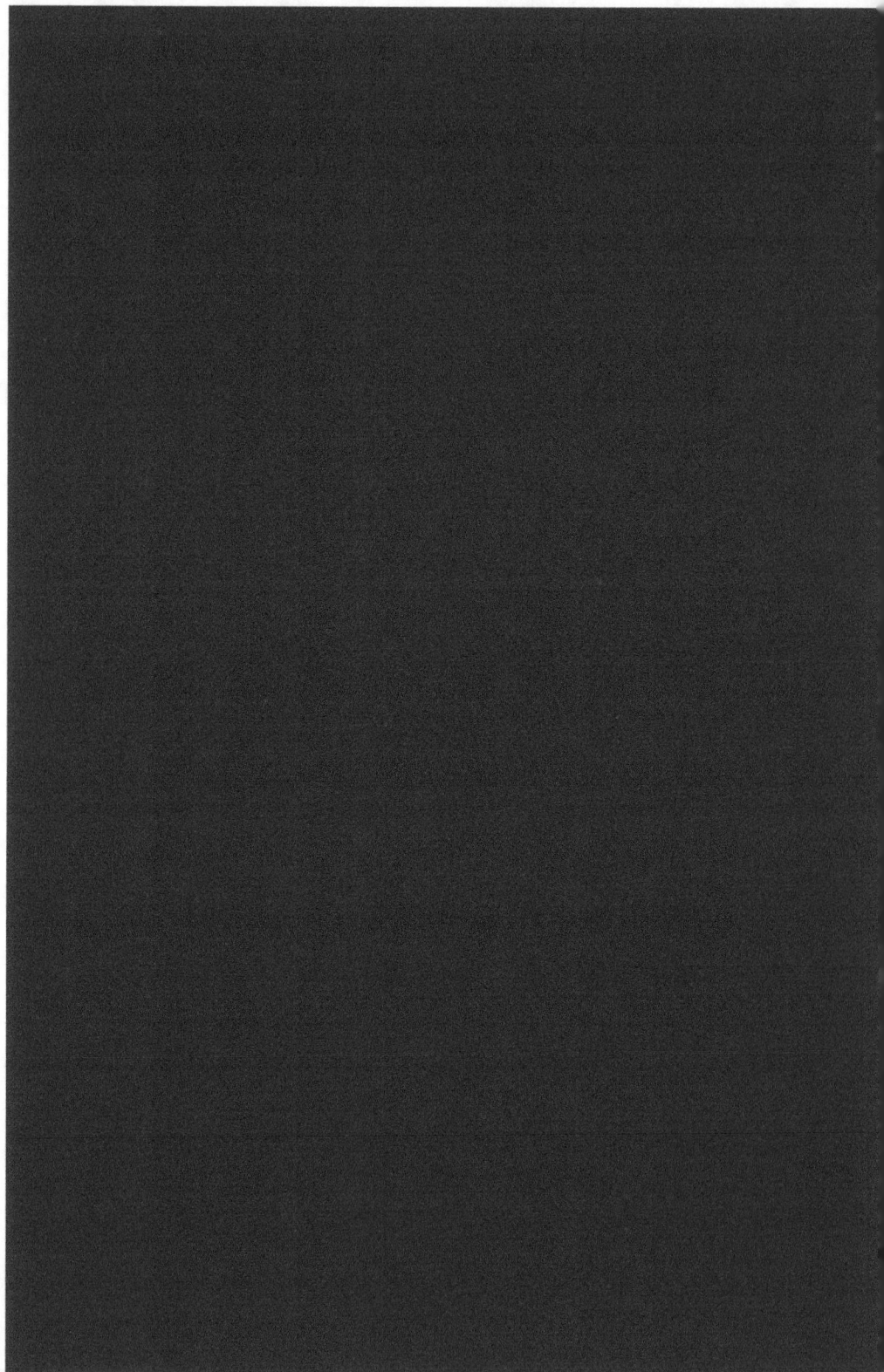

DATE _____   S   M   T   W   T   F   S

MORNING THOUGHTS & FEELINGS

_____

_____

_____

_____

_____

MORNING MEAL @ _____

I ATE:

_____

_____

I DRANK:

_____

I FELT:

_____

2-3 HOURS LATER I FELT:

_____

MID MORNING SNACK @ _____

I ATE:

_____

_____

I DRANK:

_____

I FELT:

_____

AFTERNOON MEAL @ _____

I ATE:

_____
_____

I DRANK:

_____

I FELT:

_____

2-3 HOURS LATER I FELT:

_____

AFTERNOON SNACK @ _____

I ATE:

_____
_____

I DRANK:

_____

I FELT:

_____

EVENING MEAL @ _____

I ATE:

_____
_____

I DRANK:

_____

I FELT:

_____

2-3 HOURS LATER I FELT:

_____

HAPPINESS TRACKER - ON A SCALE OF 1-5

Rate the areas below from 1-5, with 1 being least happy & 5 being most happy. Pay close attention to any trends you begin to notice regarding how the things you eat & drink affect the way you feel & your overall happiness.

My morning energy level ○ ○ ○ ○ ○

My afternoon energy level ○ ○ ○ ○ ○

My evening energy level ○ ○ ○ ○ ○

How my body feels ○ ○ ○ ○ ○

My mental clarity ○ ○ ○ ○ ○

My emotional stability ○ ○ ○ ○ ○

My excitement about life ○ ○ ○ ○ ○

My personal relationships ○ ○ ○ ○ ○

My professional relationships ○ ○ ○ ○ ○

My poop ○ ○ ○ ○ ○

EVENING THOUGHTS & FEELINGS

_____

_____

_____

_____

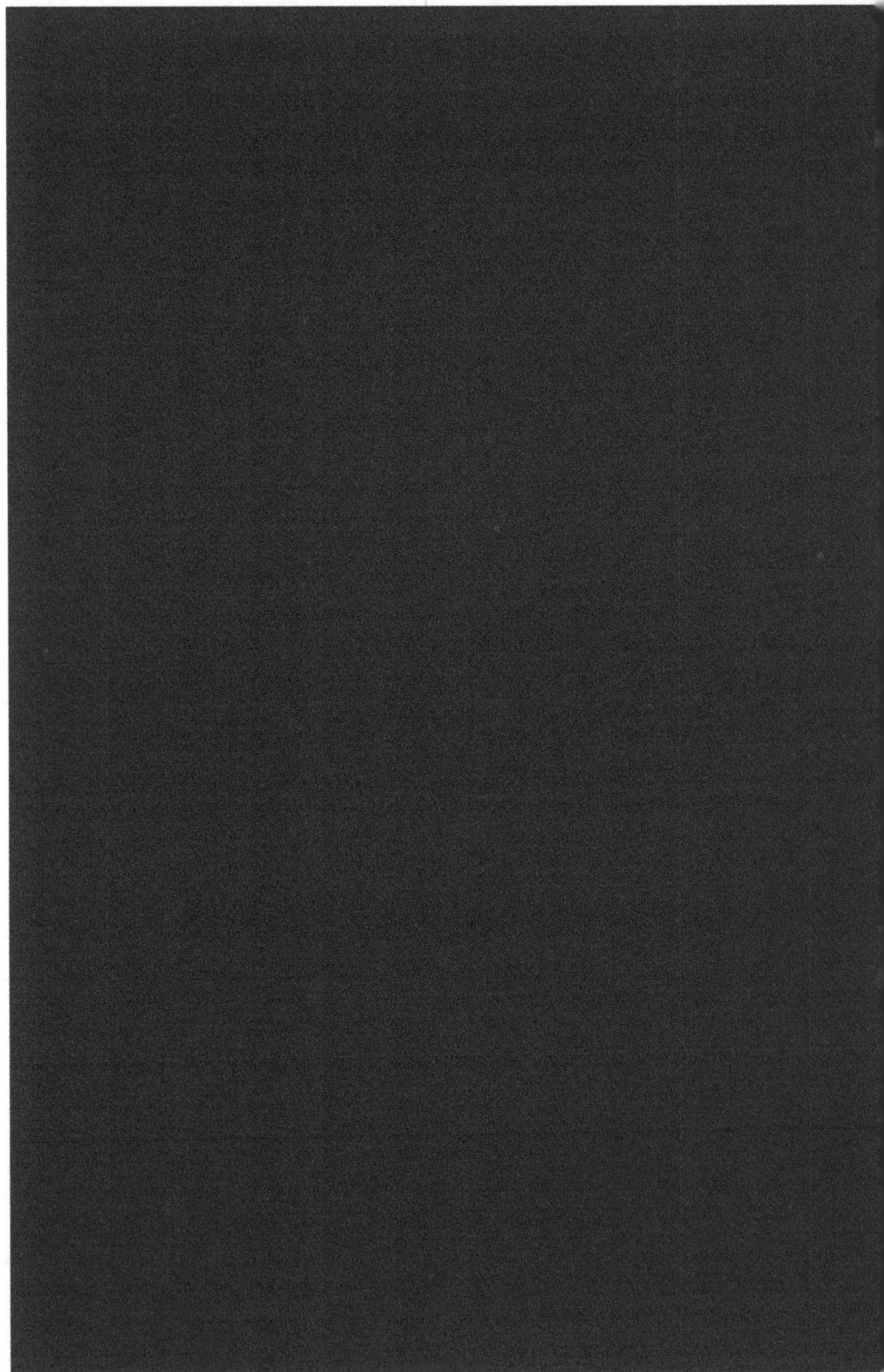

Day 27

DATE _____ S M T W T F S

MORNING THOUGHTS & FEELINGS

_____
_____
_____
_____

MORNING MEAL @ _____

I ATE:
_____
_____

I DRANK:
_____

I FELT:
_____

2-3 HOURS LATER I FELT:
_____

MID MORNING SNACK @ _____

I ATE:
_____
_____

I DRANK:
_____

I FELT:
_____

AFTERNOON MEAL @ _____

I ATE:

_____

_____

I DRANK:

_____

I FELT:

_____

2-3 HOURS LATER I FELT:

_____

AFTERNOON SNACK @ _____

I ATE:

_____

_____

I DRANK:

_____

I FELT:

_____

EVENING MEAL @ _____

I ATE:

_____

_____

I DRANK:

_____

I FELT:

_____

2-3 HOURS LATER I FELT:

_____

HAPPINESS TRACKER - ON A SCALE OF 1-5

Rate the areas below from 1-5, with 1 being least happy & 5 being most happy. Pay close attention to any trends you begin to notice regarding how the things you eat & drink affect the way you feel & your overall happiness.

My morning energy level ○ ○ ○ ○ ○

My afternoon energy level ○ ○ ○ ○ ○

My evening energy level ○ ○ ○ ○ ○

How my body feels ○ ○ ○ ○ ○

My mental clarity ○ ○ ○ ○ ○

My emotional stability ○ ○ ○ ○ ○

My excitement about life ○ ○ ○ ○ ○

My personal relationships ○ ○ ○ ○ ○

My professional relationships ○ ○ ○ ○ ○

My poop ○ ○ ○ ○ ○

EVENING THOUGHTS & FEELINGS

_____

_____

_____

_____

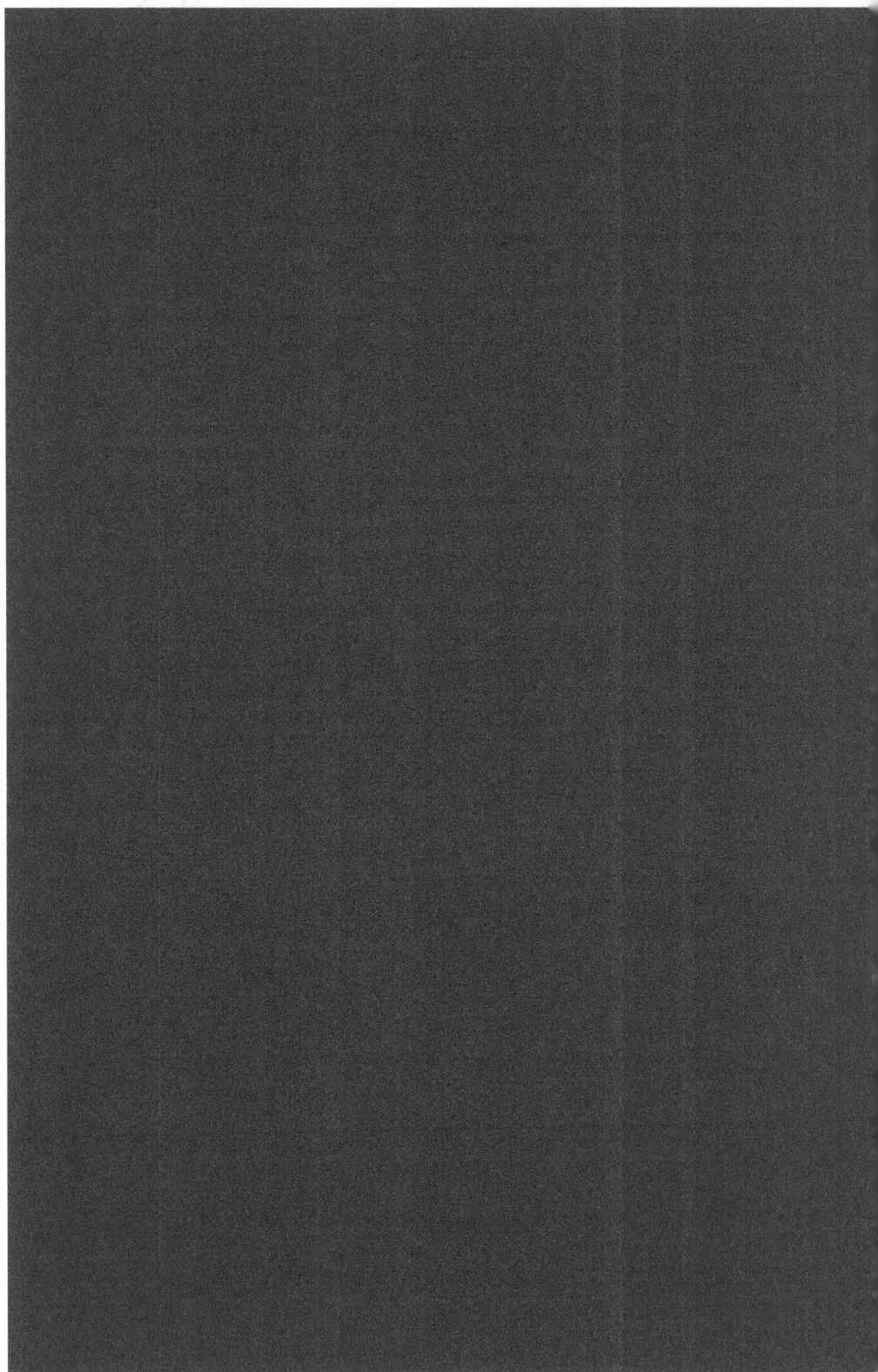

DATE   S M T W T F S

MORNING THOUGHTS & FEELINGS

_____
_____
_____
_____
_____

MORNING MEAL @ _____

I ATE:
_____
_____

I DRANK:
_____

I FELT:
_____

2-3 HOURS LATER I FELT:
_____

MID MORNING SNACK @ _____

I ATE:
_____
_____

I DRANK:
_____

I FELT:
_____

AFTERNOON MEAL @ _____

I ATE:

_____

_____

I DRANK:

_____

I FELT:

_____

2-3 HOURS LATER I FELT:

_____

AFTERNOON SNACK @ _____

I ATE:

_____

_____

I DRANK:

_____

I FELT:

_____

EVENING MEAL @ _____

I ATE:

_____

_____

I DRANK:

_____

I FELT:

_____

2-3 HOURS LATER I FELT:

_____

HAPPINESS TRACKER - ON A SCALE OF 1-5

Rate the areas below from 1-5, with 1 being least happy & 5 being most happy. Pay close attention to any trends you begin to notice regarding how the things you eat & drink affect the way you feel & your overall happiness.

My morning energy level   ○ ○ ○ ○ ○

My afternoon energy level   ○ ○ ○ ○ ○

My evening energy level   ○ ○ ○ ○ ○

How my body feels   ○ ○ ○ ○ ○

My mental clarity   ○ ○ ○ ○ ○

My emotional stability   ○ ○ ○ ○ ○

My excitement about life   ○ ○ ○ ○ ○

My personal relationships   ○ ○ ○ ○ ○

My professional relationships   ○ ○ ○ ○ ○

My poop   ○ ○ ○ ○ ○

EVENING THOUGHTS & FEELINGS

_____

_____

_____

_____

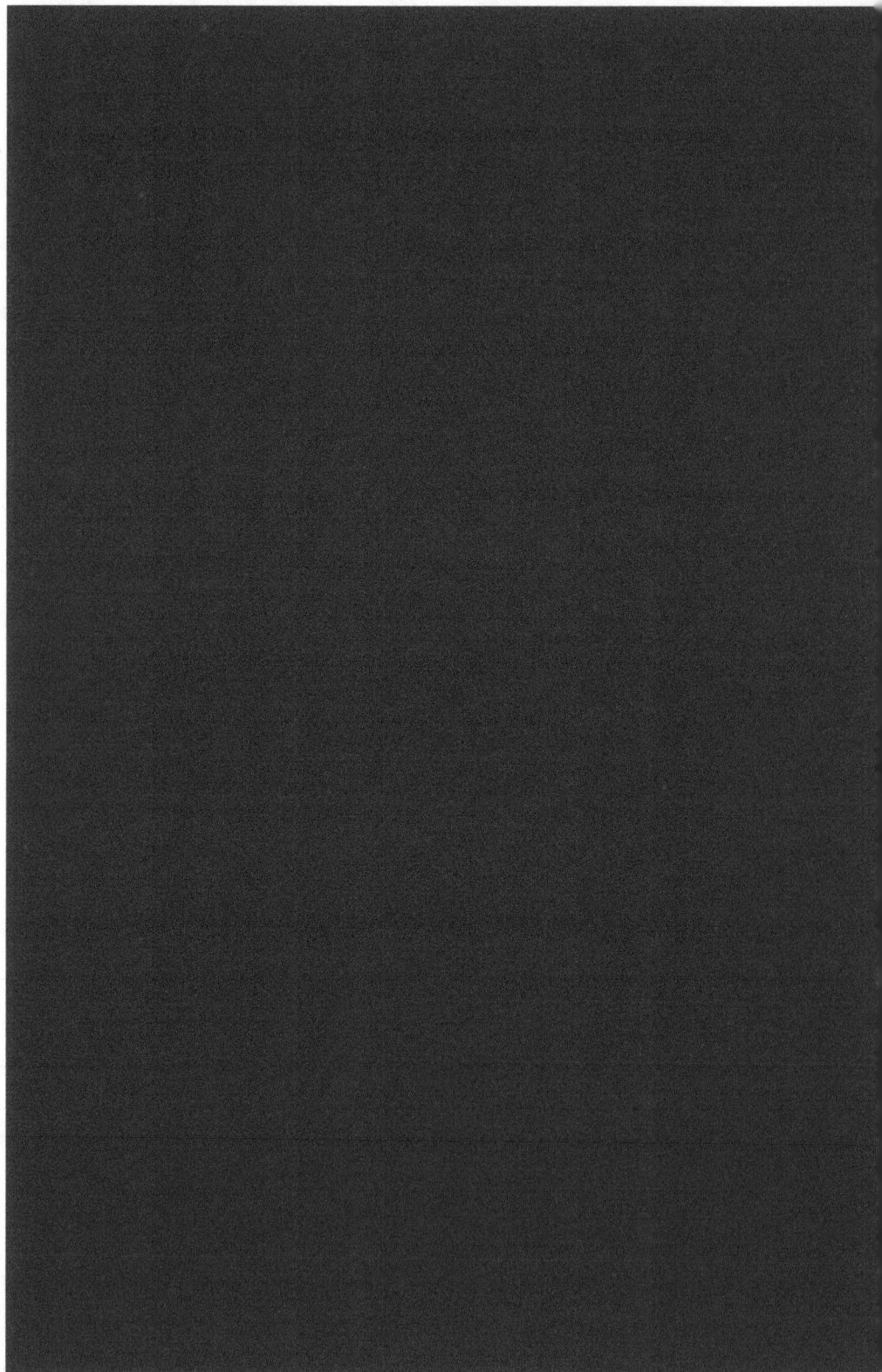

Well done!

You did it!

That's 4 weeks of tracking your happiness & eating habits.

Are you beginning to notice a trend in how you're feeling at certain times of day?

How about how you're feeling after eating certain foods?

What choices have been leaving you feeling the most happy?

How are you treating yourself?

Whether your idea of self-care is getting creative with clay, playing a board game, or going ax throwing - Treat yourself!

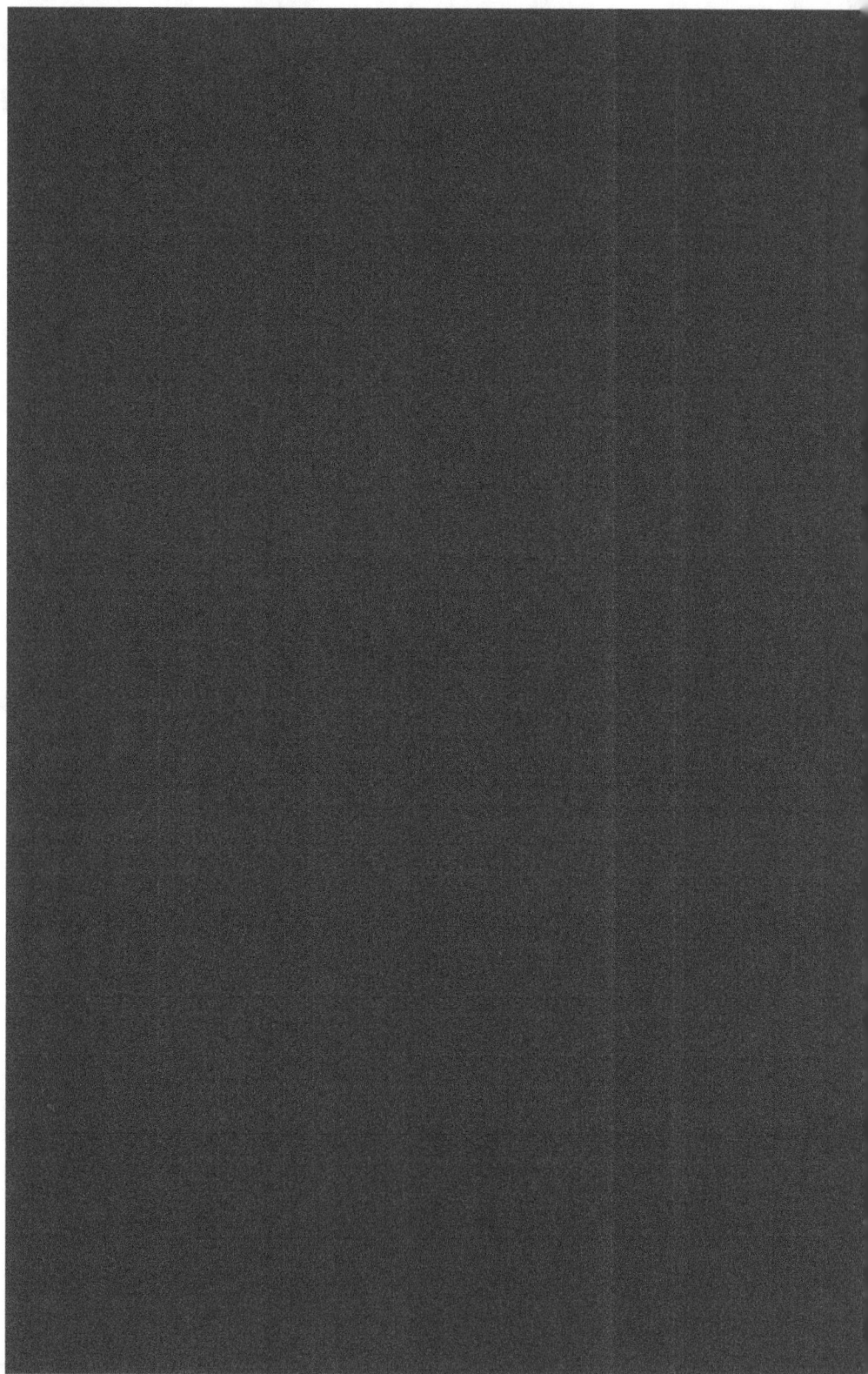

DATE _____   **S M T W T F S**

MORNING THOUGHTS & FEELINGS

_____
_____
_____
_____

MORNING MEAL @ _____

I ATE:

_____
_____

I DRANK:

_____

I FELT:

_____

2-3 HOURS LATER I FELT:

_____

MID MORNING SNACK @ _____

I ATE:

_____
_____

I DRANK:

_____

I FELT:

_____

AFTERNOON MEAL @ _____

I ATE:

_____

_____

I DRANK:

_____

I FELT:

_____

2-3 HOURS LATER I FELT:

_____

AFTERNOON SNACK @ _____

I ATE:

_____

_____

I DRANK:

_____

I FELT:

_____

EVENING MEAL @ _____

I ATE:

_____

_____

I DRANK:

_____

I FELT:

_____

2-3 HOURS LATER I FELT:

_____

HAPPINESS TRACKER - ON A SCALE OF 1-5

Rate the areas below from 1-5, with 1 being least happy & 5 being most happy. Pay close attention to any trends you begin to notice regarding how the things you eat & drink affect the way you feel & your overall happiness.

My morning energy level	○	○	○	○	○
My afternoon energy level	○	○	○	○	○
My evening energy level	○	○	○	○	○
How my body feels	○	○	○	○	○
My mental clarity	○	○	○	○	○
My emotional stability	○	○	○	○	○
My excitement about life	○	○	○	○	○
My personal relationships	○	○	○	○	○
My professional relationships	○	○	○	○	○
My poop	○	○	○	○	○

EVENING THOUGHTS & FEELINGS

_____

_____

_____

_____

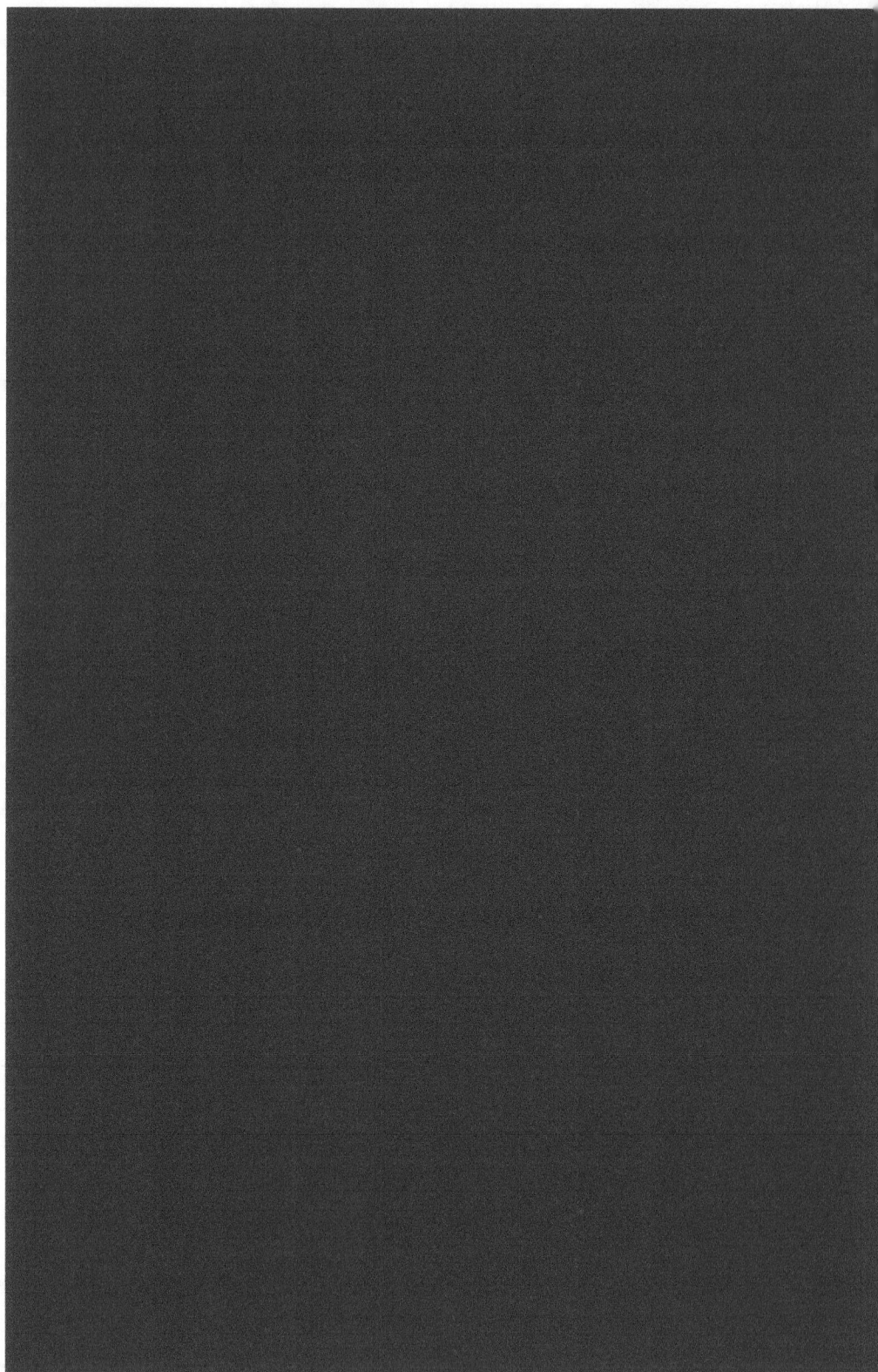

DATE _____   S   M   T   W   T   F   S

MORNING THOUGHTS & FEELINGS

_____
_____
_____
_____
_____

MORNING MEAL @ _____

I ATE:

_____
_____

I DRANK:

_____

I FELT:

_____

2-3 HOURS LATER I FELT:

_____

MID MORNING SNACK @ _____

I ATE:

_____
_____

I DRANK:

_____

I FELT:

_____

AFTERNOON MEAL @ _____

I ATE:

_____
_____

I DRANK:

_____

I FELT:

_____

2-3 HOURS LATER I FELT:

_____

AFTERNOON SNACK @ _____

I ATE:

_____
_____

I DRANK:

_____

I FELT:

_____

EVENING MEAL @ _____

I ATE:

_____
_____

I DRANK:

_____

I FELT:

_____

2-3 HOURS LATER I FELT:

_____

HAPPINESS TRACKER - ON A SCALE OF 1-5

Rate the areas below from 1-5, with 1 being least happy & 5 being most happy. Pay close attention to any trends you begin to notice regarding how the things you eat & drink affect the way you feel & your overall happiness.

My morning energy level	○	○	○	○	○
My afternoon energy level	○	○	○	○	○
My evening energy level	○	○	○	○	○
How my body feels	○	○	○	○	○
My mental clarity	○	○	○	○	○
My emotional stability	○	○	○	○	○
My excitement about life	○	○	○	○	○
My personal relationships	○	○	○	○	○
My professional relationships	○	○	○	○	○
My poop	○	○	○	○	○

EVENING THOUGHTS & FEELINGS

_____

_____

_____

_____

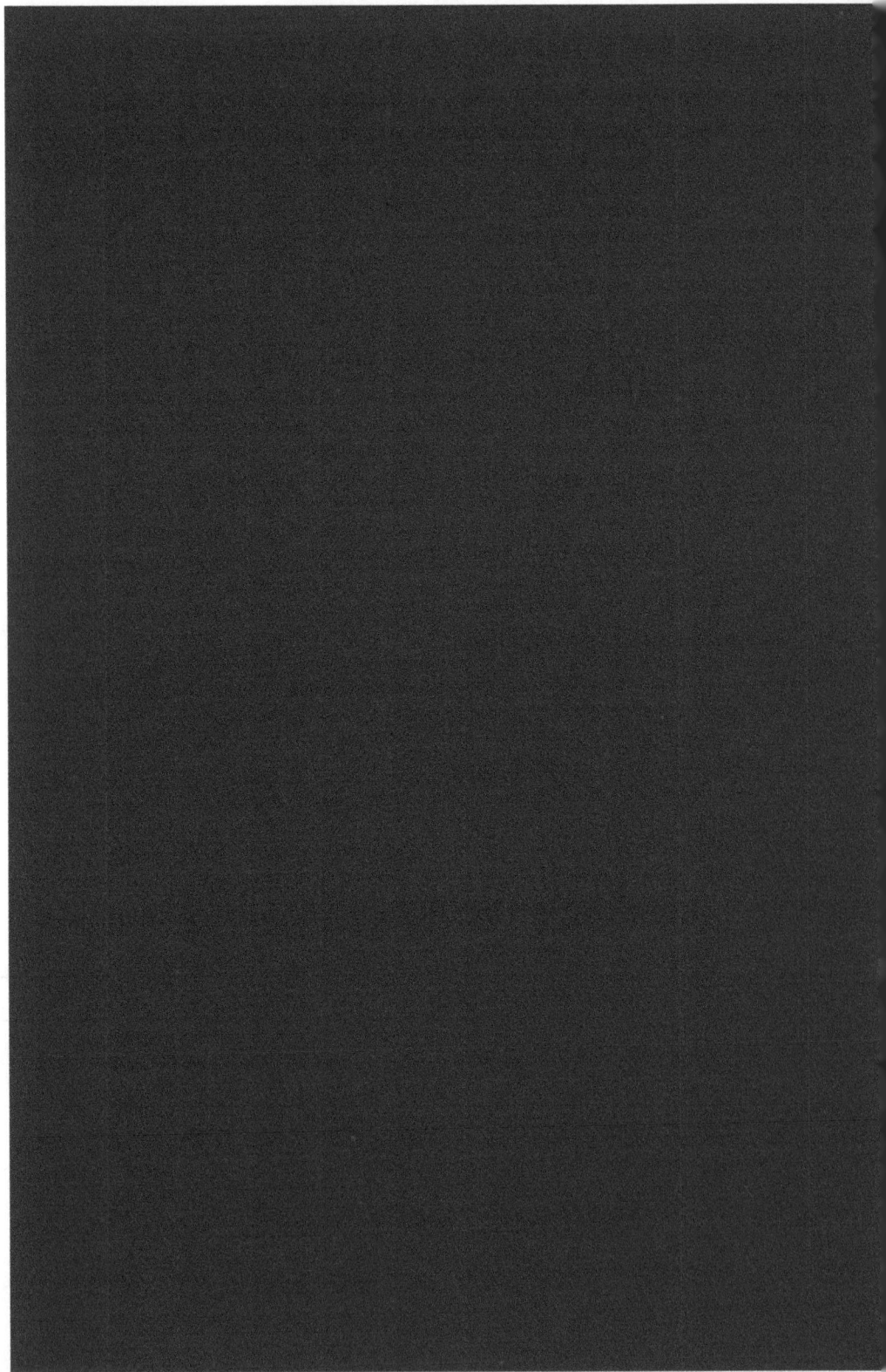

Day 31

DATE   S   M   T   W   T   F   S

MORNING THOUGHTS & FEELINGS

_____
_____
_____
_____
_____

MORNING MEAL @ _____

I ATE:
_____
_____

I DRANK:
_____

I FELT:
_____

2-3 HOURS LATER I FELT:
_____

MID MORNING SNACK @ _____

I ATE:
_____
_____

I DRANK:
_____

I FELT:
_____

AFTERNOON MEAL @ _____

I ATE:

_____

_____

I DRANK:

_____

I FELT:

_____

2-3 HOURS LATER I FELT:

_____

AFTERNOON SNACK @ _____

I ATE:

_____

_____

I DRANK:

_____

I FELT:

_____

EVENING MEAL @ _____

I ATE:

_____

_____

I DRANK:

_____

I FELT:

_____

2-3 HOURS LATER I FELT:

_____

HAPPINESS TRACKER - ON A SCALE OF 1-5

Rate the areas below from 1-5, with 1 being least happy & 5 being most happy. Pay close attention to any trends you begin to notice regarding how the things you eat & drink affect the way you feel & your overall happiness.

My morning energy level   ○ ○ ○ ○ ○

My afternoon energy level   ○ ○ ○ ○ ○

My evening energy level   ○ ○ ○ ○ ○

How my body feels   ○ ○ ○ ○ ○

My mental clarity   ○ ○ ○ ○ ○

My emotional stability   ○ ○ ○ ○ ○

My excitement about life   ○ ○ ○ ○ ○

My personal relationships   ○ ○ ○ ○ ○

My professional relationships   ○ ○ ○ ○ ○

My poop   ○ ○ ○ ○ ○

EVENING THOUGHTS & FEELINGS

_____

_____

_____

_____

DATE _____   S M T W T F S

MORNING THOUGHTS & FEELINGS

_____
_____
_____
_____

MORNING MEAL @ _____

I ATE:
_____
_____

I DRANK:
_____

I FELT:
_____

2-3 HOURS LATER I FELT:
_____

MID MORNING SNACK @ _____

I ATE:
_____
_____

I DRANK:
_____

I FELT:
_____

AFTERNOON MEAL @ _____

I ATE:

_____
_____

I DRANK:

_____

I FELT:

_____

2-3 HOURS LATER I FELT:

_____

AFTERNOON SNACK @ _____

I ATE:

_____
_____

I DRANK:

_____

I FELT:

_____

EVENING MEAL @ _____

I ATE:

_____
_____
_____

I DRANK:

_____

I FELT:

_____

2-3 HOURS LATER I FELT:

_____

HAPPINESS TRACKER - ON A SCALE OF 1-5

Rate the areas below from 1-5, with 1 being least happy & 5 being most happy. Pay close attention to any trends you begin to notice regarding how the things you eat & drink affect the way you feel & your overall happiness.

My morning energy level ○ ○ ○ ○ ○

My afternoon energy level ○ ○ ○ ○ ○

My evening energy level ○ ○ ○ ○ ○

How my body feels ○ ○ ○ ○ ○

My mental clarity ○ ○ ○ ○ ○

My emotional stability ○ ○ ○ ○ ○

My excitement about life ○ ○ ○ ○ ○

My personal relationships ○ ○ ○ ○ ○

My professional relationships ○ ○ ○ ○ ○

My poop ○ ○ ○ ○ ○

EVENING THOUGHTS & FEELINGS

_____

_____

_____

_____

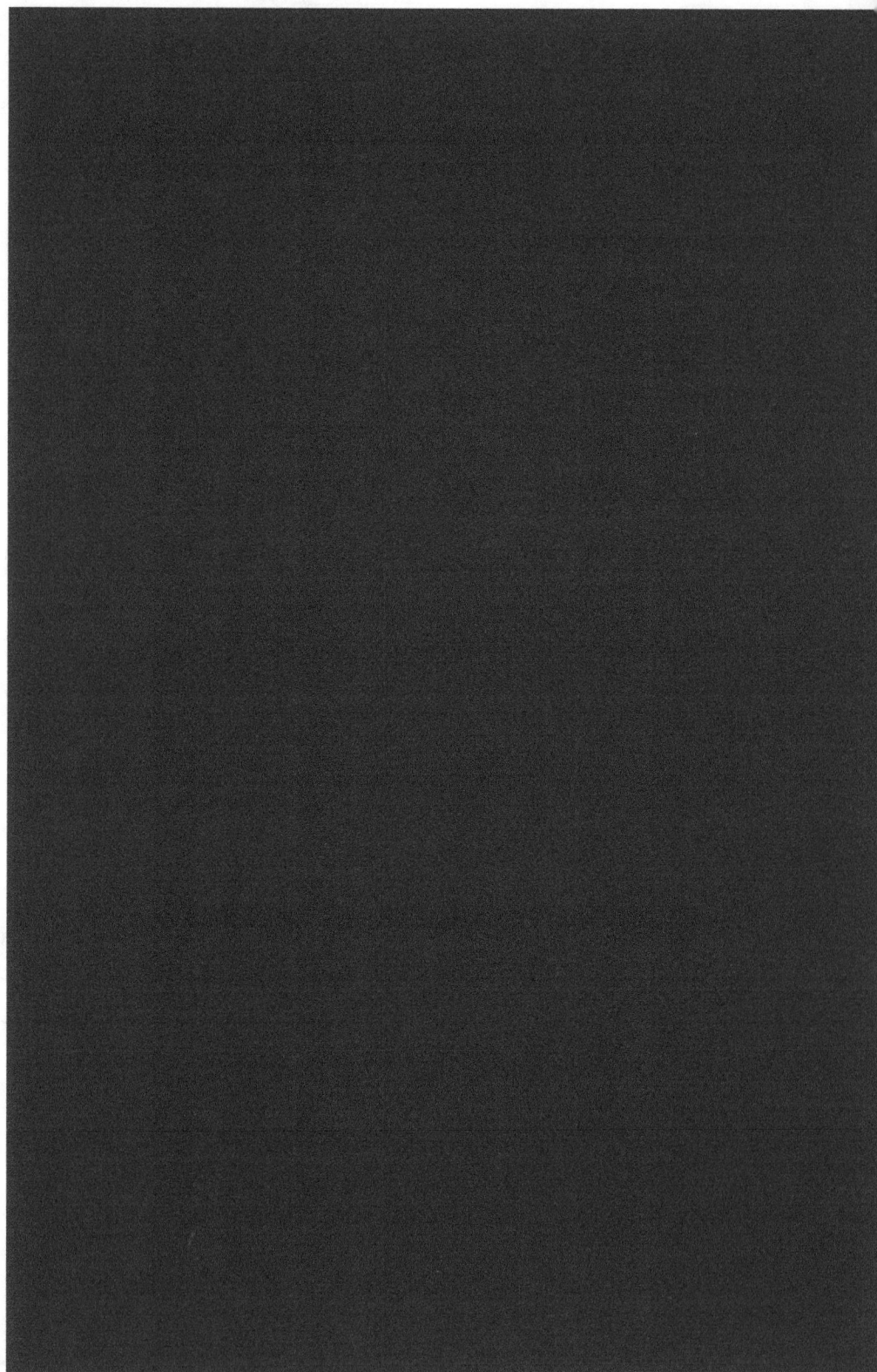

DATE   S   M   T   W   T   F   S

MORNING THOUGHTS & FEELINGS

_____
_____
_____
_____

MORNING MEAL @ _____

I ATE:
_____
_____

I DRANK:
_____

I FELT:
_____

2-3 HOURS LATER I FELT:
_____

MID MORNING SNACK @ _____

I ATE:
_____
_____

I DRANK:
_____

I FELT:
_____

AFTERNOON MEAL @ _____

I ATE:

_____

_____

I DRANK:

_____

I FELT:

_____

2-3 HOURS LATER I FELT:

_____

AFTERNOON SNACK @ _____

I ATE:

_____

_____

I DRANK:

_____

I FELT:

_____

EVENING MEAL @ _____

I ATE:

_____

_____

_____

I DRANK:

_____

I FELT:

_____

2-3 HOURS LATER I FELT:

_____

HAPPINESS TRACKER - ON A SCALE OF 1-5

Rate the areas below from 1-5, with 1 being least happy & 5 being most happy. Pay close attention to any trends you begin to notice regarding how the things you eat & drink affect the way you feel & your overall happiness.

My morning energy level   ○ ○ ○ ○ ○

My afternoon energy level   ○ ○ ○ ○ ○

My evening energy level   ○ ○ ○ ○ ○

How my body feels   ○ ○ ○ ○ ○

My mental clarity   ○ ○ ○ ○ ○

My emotional stability   ○ ○ ○ ○ ○

My excitement about life   ○ ○ ○ ○ ○

My personal relationships   ○ ○ ○ ○ ○

My professional relationships   ○ ○ ○ ○ ○

My poop   ○ ○ ○ ○ ○

EVENING THOUGHTS & FEELINGS

_____

_____

_____

_____

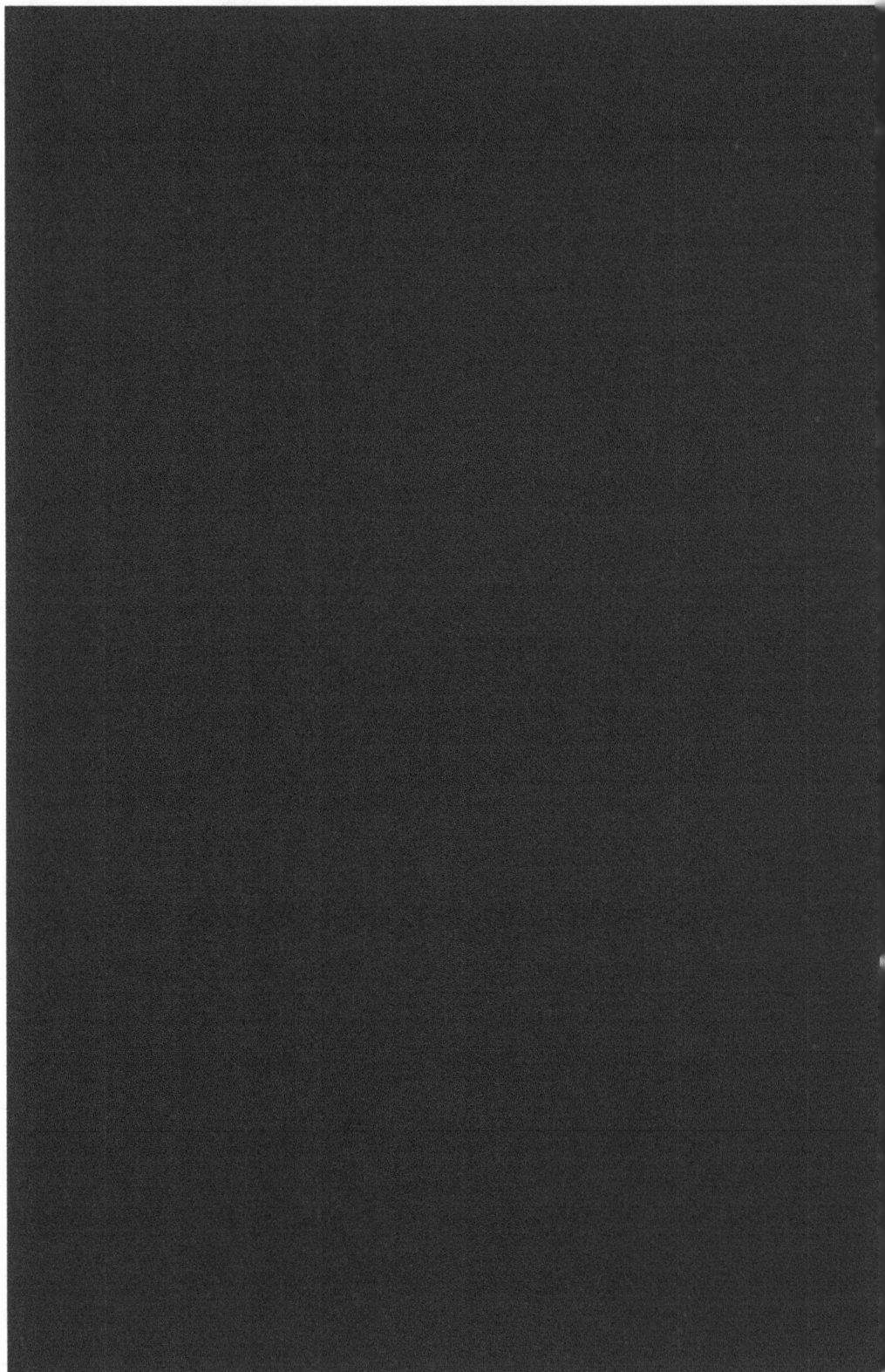

DATE _____   S   M   T   W   T   F   S

MORNING THOUGHTS & FEELINGS

_____
_____
_____
_____
_____

MORNING MEAL @ _____

I ATE:
_____
_____

I DRANK:
_____

I FELT:
_____

2-3 HOURS LATER I FELT:
_____

MID MORNING SNACK @ _____

I ATE:
_____
_____

I DRANK:
_____

I FELT:
_____

AFTERNOON MEAL @ _____

I ATE:

_____
_____

I DRANK:

_____

I FELT:

_____

2-3 HOURS LATER I FELT:

_____

AFTERNOON SNACK @ _____

I ATE:

_____
_____

I DRANK:

_____

I FELT:

_____

EVENING MEAL @ _____

I ATE:

_____
_____

I DRANK:

_____

I FELT:

_____

2-3 HOURS LATER I FELT:

_____

HAPPINESS TRACKER - ON A SCALE OF 1-5

Rate the areas below from 1-5, with 1 being least happy & 5 being most happy. Pay close attention to any trends you begin to notice regarding how the things you eat & drink affect the way you feel & your overall happiness.

My morning energy level	○ ○ ○ ○ ○
My afternoon energy level	○ ○ ○ ○ ○
My evening energy level	○ ○ ○ ○ ○
How my body feels	○ ○ ○ ○ ○
My mental clarity	○ ○ ○ ○ ○
My emotional stability	○ ○ ○ ○ ○
My excitement about life	○ ○ ○ ○ ○
My personal relationships	○ ○ ○ ○ ○
My professional relationships	○ ○ ○ ○ ○
My poop	○ ○ ○ ○ ○

EVENING THOUGHTS & FEELINGS

_____

_____

_____

_____

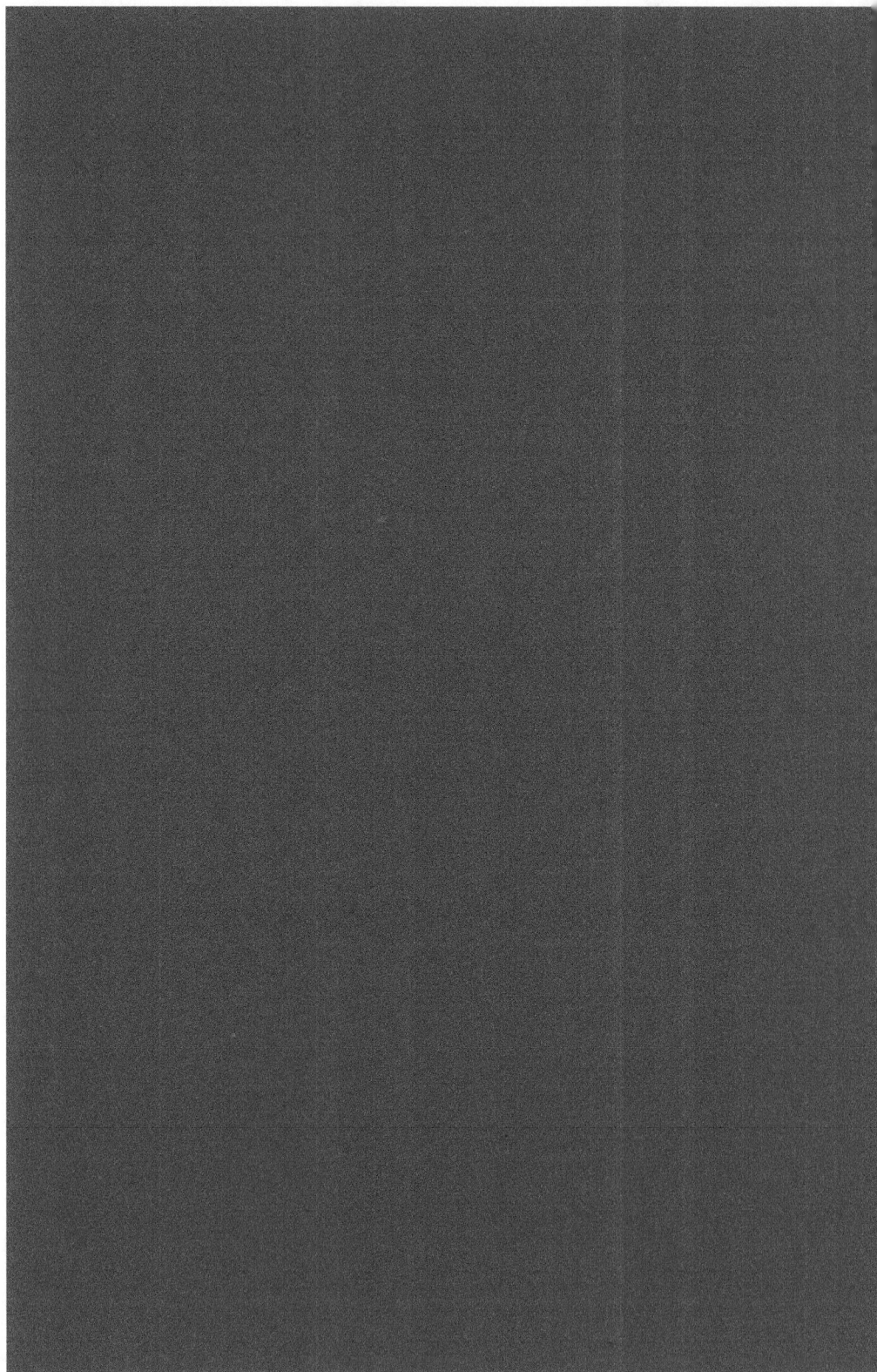

Day 35

DATE _____   S M T W T F S

MORNING THOUGHTS & FEELINGS

_____
_____
_____
_____
_____

MORNING MEAL @ _____

I ATE:
_____
_____

I DRANK:
_____

I FELT:
_____

2-3 HOURS LATER I FELT:
_____

MID MORNING SNACK @ _____

I ATE:
_____
_____

I DRANK:
_____

I FELT:
_____

AFTERNOON MEAL @ _____

I ATE:

_____

_____

I DRANK:

_____

I FELT:

_____

2-3 HOURS LATER I FELT:

_____

AFTERNOON SNACK @ _____

I ATE:

_____

_____

I DRANK:

_____

I FELT:

_____

EVENING MEAL @ _____

I ATE:

_____

_____

I DRANK:

_____

I FELT:

_____

2-3 HOURS LATER I FELT:

_____

HAPPINESS TRACKER - ON A SCALE OF 1-5

Rate the areas below from 1-5, with 1 being least happy & 5 being most happy. Pay close attention to any trends you begin to notice regarding how the things you eat & drink affect the way you feel & your overall happiness.

My morning energy level   ○ ○ ○ ○ ○

My afternoon energy level   ○ ○ ○ ○ ○

My evening energy level   ○ ○ ○ ○ ○

How my body feels   ○ ○ ○ ○ ○

My mental clarity   ○ ○ ○ ○ ○

My emotional stability   ○ ○ ○ ○ ○

My excitement about life   ○ ○ ○ ○ ○

My personal relationships   ○ ○ ○ ○ ○

My professional relationships   ○ ○ ○ ○ ○

My poop   ○ ○ ○ ○ ○

EVENING THOUGHTS & FEELINGS

_____

_____

_____

_____

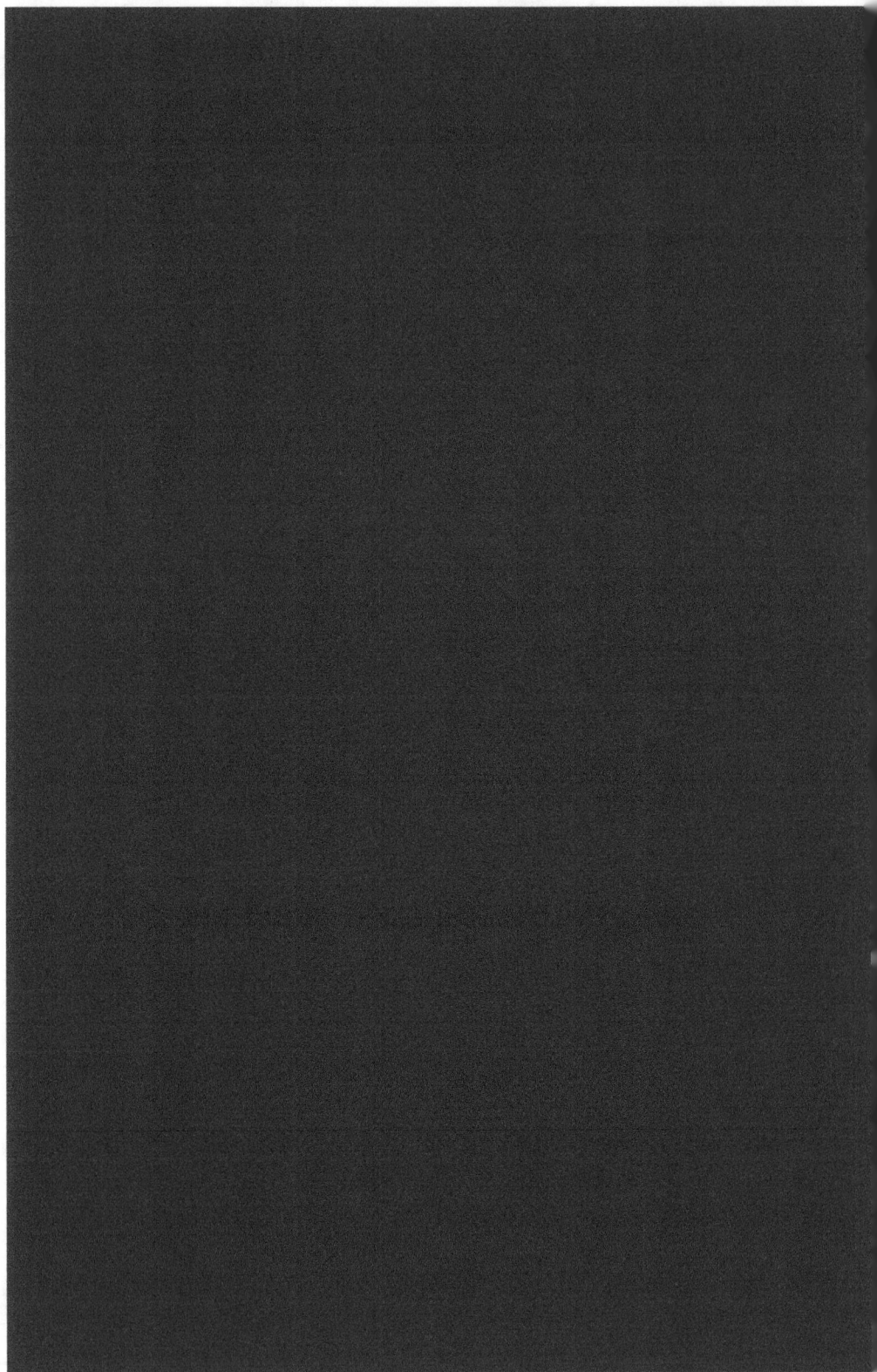

Well done!

You did it!

That's 5 weeks - 35 days - of eating
intuitively & tracking your happiness

Have you noticed any trends in what
you're eating & how you're feeling?

It's important to recognize &
appreciate the amazing progress
you're making every single day.

How are you treating yourself?

Whether your idea of self-care is
unplugging & getting lost in the
woods or relaxing with yoga &
meditation - Treat yourself!

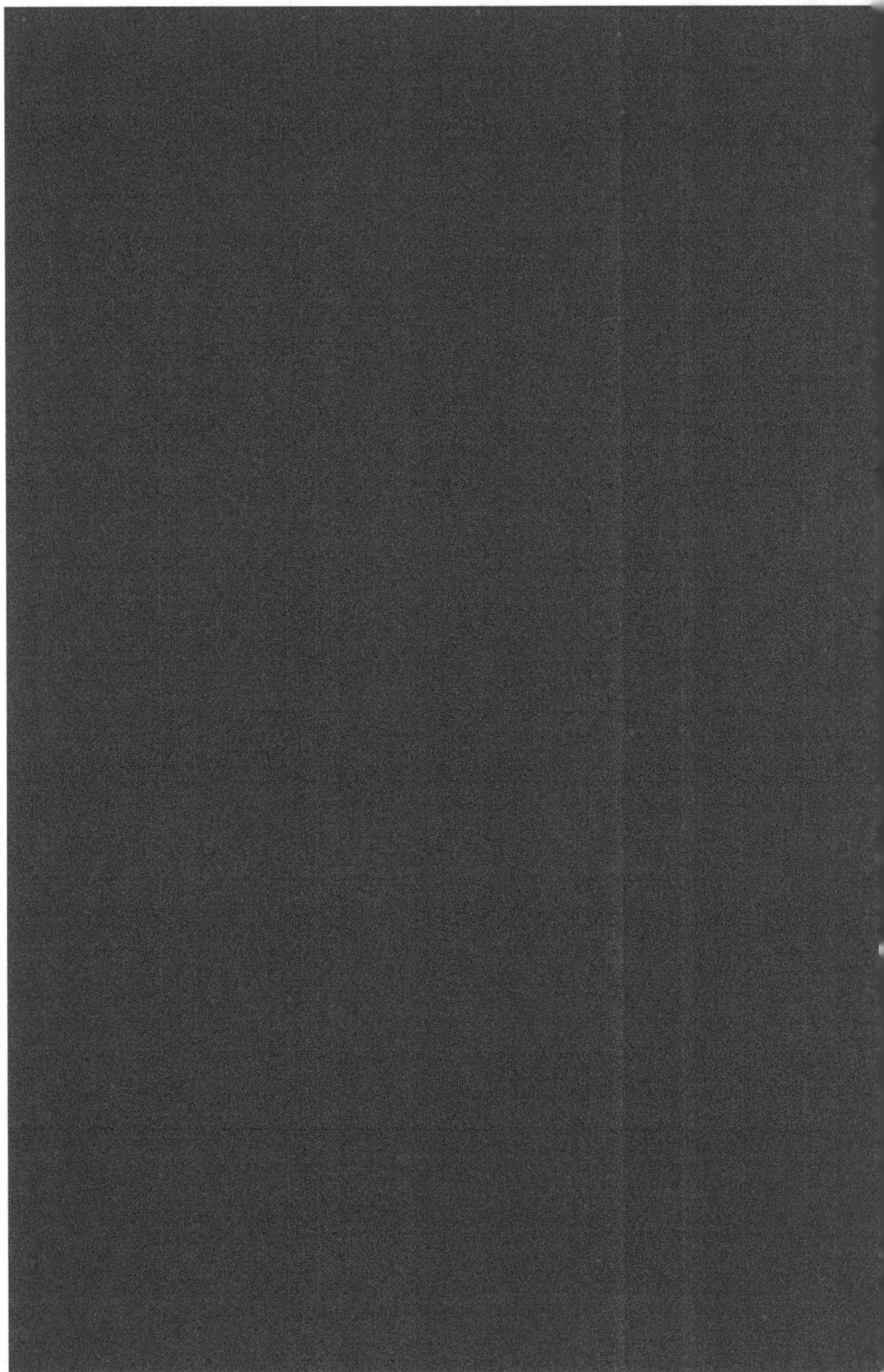

DATE _____   **S M T W T F S**

MORNING THOUGHTS & FEELINGS

_____

_____

_____

_____

MORNING MEAL @ _____

I ATE:

_____

_____

I DRANK:

_____

I FELT:

_____

2-3 HOURS LATER I FELT:

_____

MID MORNING SNACK @ _____

I ATE:

_____

_____

I DRANK:

_____

I FELT:

_____

AFTERNOON MEAL @ _____

I ATE:

_____

_____

I DRANK:

_____

I FELT:

_____

2-3 HOURS LATER I FELT:

_____

AFTERNOON SNACK @ _____

I ATE:

_____

_____

I DRANK:

_____

I FELT:

_____

EVENING MEAL @ _____

I ATE:

_____

_____

I DRANK:

_____

I FELT:

_____

2-3 HOURS LATER I FELT:

_____

HAPPINESS TRACKER - ON A SCALE OF 1-5

Rate the areas below from 1-5, with 1 being least happy & 5 being most happy. Pay close attention to any trends you begin to notice regarding how the things you eat & drink affect the way you feel & your overall happiness.

My morning energy level   ○ ○ ○ ○ ○

My afternoon energy level   ○ ○ ○ ○ ○

My evening energy level   ○ ○ ○ ○ ○

How my body feels   ○ ○ ○ ○ ○

My mental clarity   ○ ○ ○ ○ ○

My emotional stability   ○ ○ ○ ○ ○

My excitement about life   ○ ○ ○ ○ ○

My personal relationships   ○ ○ ○ ○ ○

My professional relationships   ○ ○ ○ ○ ○

My poop   ○ ○ ○ ○ ○

EVENING THOUGHTS & FEELINGS

_____

_____

_____

_____

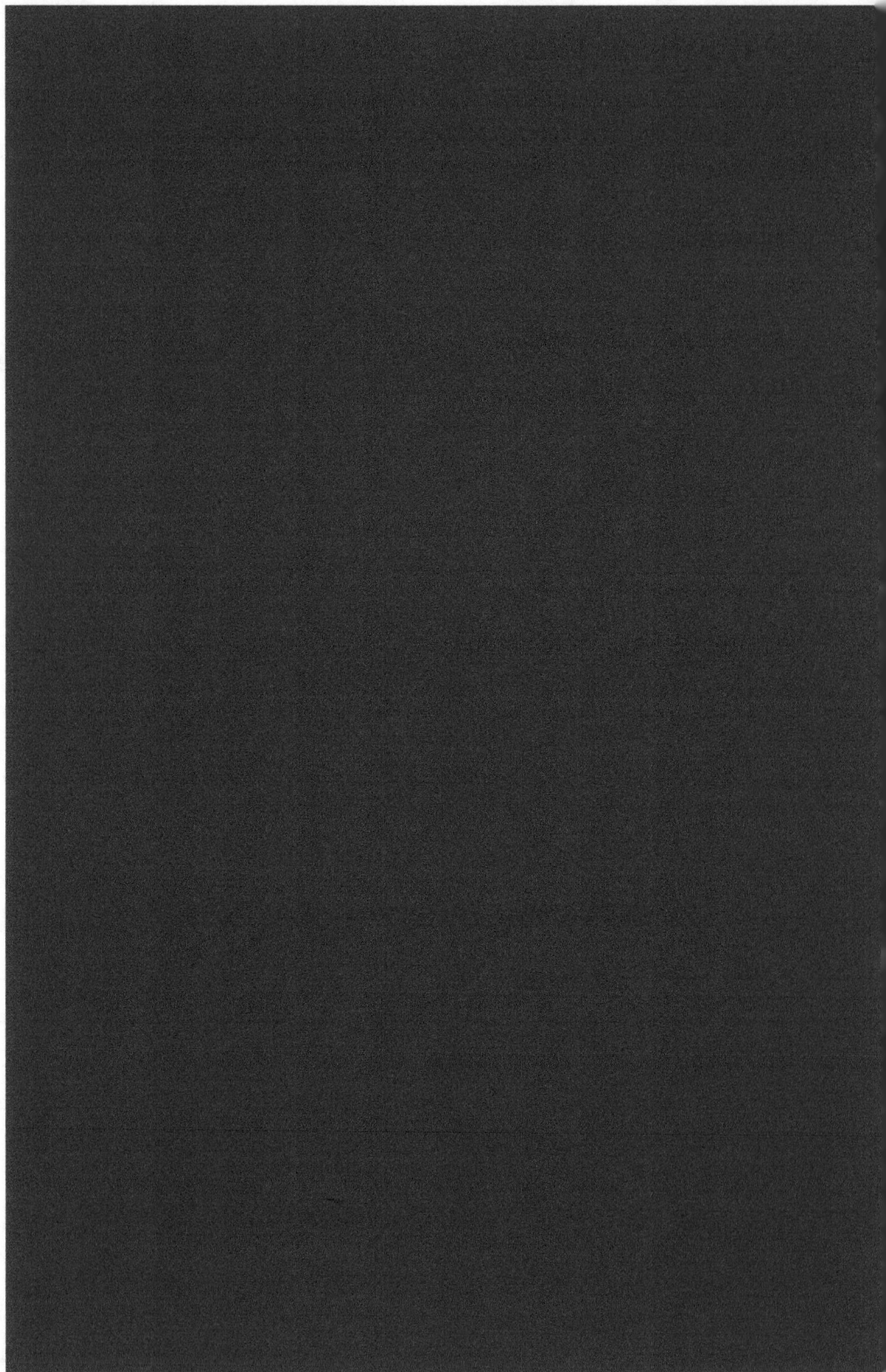

DATE _____   S M T W T F S

MORNING THOUGHTS & FEELINGS

_____
_____
_____
_____

MORNING MEAL @ _____

I ATE:
_____
_____

I DRANK:
_____

I FELT:
_____

2-3 HOURS LATER I FELT:
_____

MID MORNING SNACK @ _____

I ATE:
_____
_____

I DRANK:
_____

I FELT:
_____

AFTERNOON MEAL @ _____

I ATE:

_____

_____

I DRANK:

_____

I FELT:

_____

2-3 HOURS LATER I FELT:

_____

AFTERNOON SNACK @ _____

I ATE:

_____

_____

I DRANK:

_____

I FELT:

_____

EVENING MEAL @ _____

I ATE:

_____

_____

I DRANK:

_____

I FELT:

_____

2-3 HOURS LATER I FELT:

_____

HAPPINESS TRACKER - ON A SCALE OF 1-5

Rate the areas below from 1-5, with 1 being least happy & 5 being most happy. Pay close attention to any trends you begin to notice regarding how the things you eat & drink affect the way you feel & your overall happiness.

My morning energy level	○	○	○	○	○
My afternoon energy level	○	○	○	○	○
My evening energy level	○	○	○	○	○
How my body feels	○	○	○	○	○
My mental clarity	○	○	○	○	○
My emotional stability	○	○	○	○	○
My excitement about life	○	○	○	○	○
My personal relationships	○	○	○	○	○
My professional relationships	○	○	○	○	○
My poop	○	○	○	○	○

EVENING THOUGHTS & FEELINGS

_____

_____

_____

_____

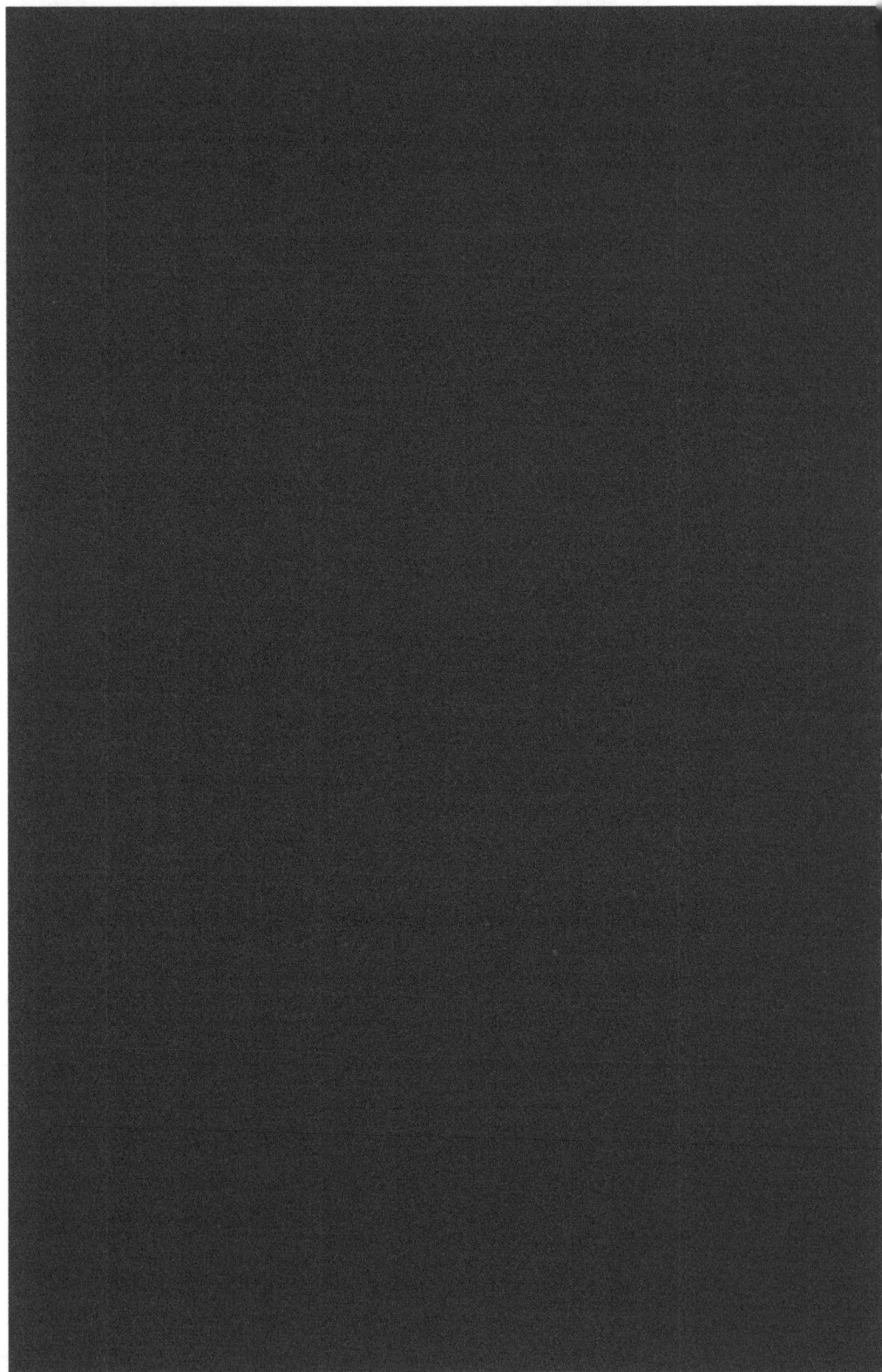

DATE **S M T W T F S**

MORNING THOUGHTS & FEELINGS

_____
_____
_____
_____
_____

MORNING MEAL @ _____

I ATE:
_____
_____

I DRANK:
_____

I FELT:
_____

2-3 HOURS LATER I FELT:
_____

MID MORNING SNACK @ _____

I ATE:
_____
_____

I DRANK:
_____

I FELT:
_____

AFTERNOON MEAL @ _____

I ATE:

_____
_____

I DRANK:

_____

I FELT:

_____

2-3 HOURS LATER I FELT:

_____

AFTERNOON SNACK @ _____

I ATE:

_____
_____

I DRANK:

_____

I FELT:

_____

EVENING MEAL @ _____

I ATE:

_____
_____

I DRANK:

_____

I FELT:

_____

2-3 HOURS LATER I FELT:

_____

HAPPINESS TRACKER - ON A SCALE OF 1-5

Rate the areas below from 1-5, with 1 being least happy & 5 being most happy. Pay close attention to any trends you begin to notice regarding how the things you eat & drink affect the way you feel & your overall happiness.

My morning energy level	○ ○ ○ ○ ○
My afternoon energy level	○ ○ ○ ○ ○
My evening energy level	○ ○ ○ ○ ○
How my body feels	○ ○ ○ ○ ○
My mental clarity	○ ○ ○ ○ ○
My emotional stability	○ ○ ○ ○ ○
My excitement about life	○ ○ ○ ○ ○
My personal relationships	○ ○ ○ ○ ○
My professional relationships	○ ○ ○ ○ ○
My poop	○ ○ ○ ○ ○

EVENING THOUGHTS & FEELINGS

_____

_____

_____

_____

DATE _____   S M T W T F S

MORNING THOUGHTS & FEELINGS

_____
_____
_____
_____

MORNING MEAL @ _____

I ATE:
_____
_____

I DRANK:
_____

I FELT:
_____

2-3 HOURS LATER I FELT:
_____

MID MORNING SNACK @ _____

I ATE:
_____
_____

I DRANK:
_____

I FELT:
_____

AFTERNOON MEAL @ _____

I ATE:

_____

_____

I DRANK:

_____

I FELT:

_____

2-3 HOURS LATER I FELT:

_____

AFTERNOON SNACK @ _____

I ATE:

_____

_____

I DRANK:

_____

I FELT:

_____

EVENING MEAL @ _____

I ATE:

_____

_____

I DRANK:

_____

I FELT:

_____

2-3 HOURS LATER I FELT:

_____

HAPPINESS TRACKER - ON A SCALE OF 1-5

Rate the areas below from 1-5, with 1 being least happy & 5 being most happy. Pay close attention to any trends you begin to notice regarding how the things you eat & drink affect the way you feel & your overall happiness.

My morning energy level ○ ○ ○ ○ ○

My afternoon energy level ○ ○ ○ ○ ○

My evening energy level ○ ○ ○ ○ ○

How my body feels ○ ○ ○ ○ ○

My mental clarity ○ ○ ○ ○ ○

My emotional stability ○ ○ ○ ○ ○

My excitement about life ○ ○ ○ ○ ○

My personal relationships ○ ○ ○ ○ ○

My professional relationships ○ ○ ○ ○ ○

My poop ○ ○ ○ ○ ○

EVENING THOUGHTS & FEELINGS

_____

_____

_____

_____

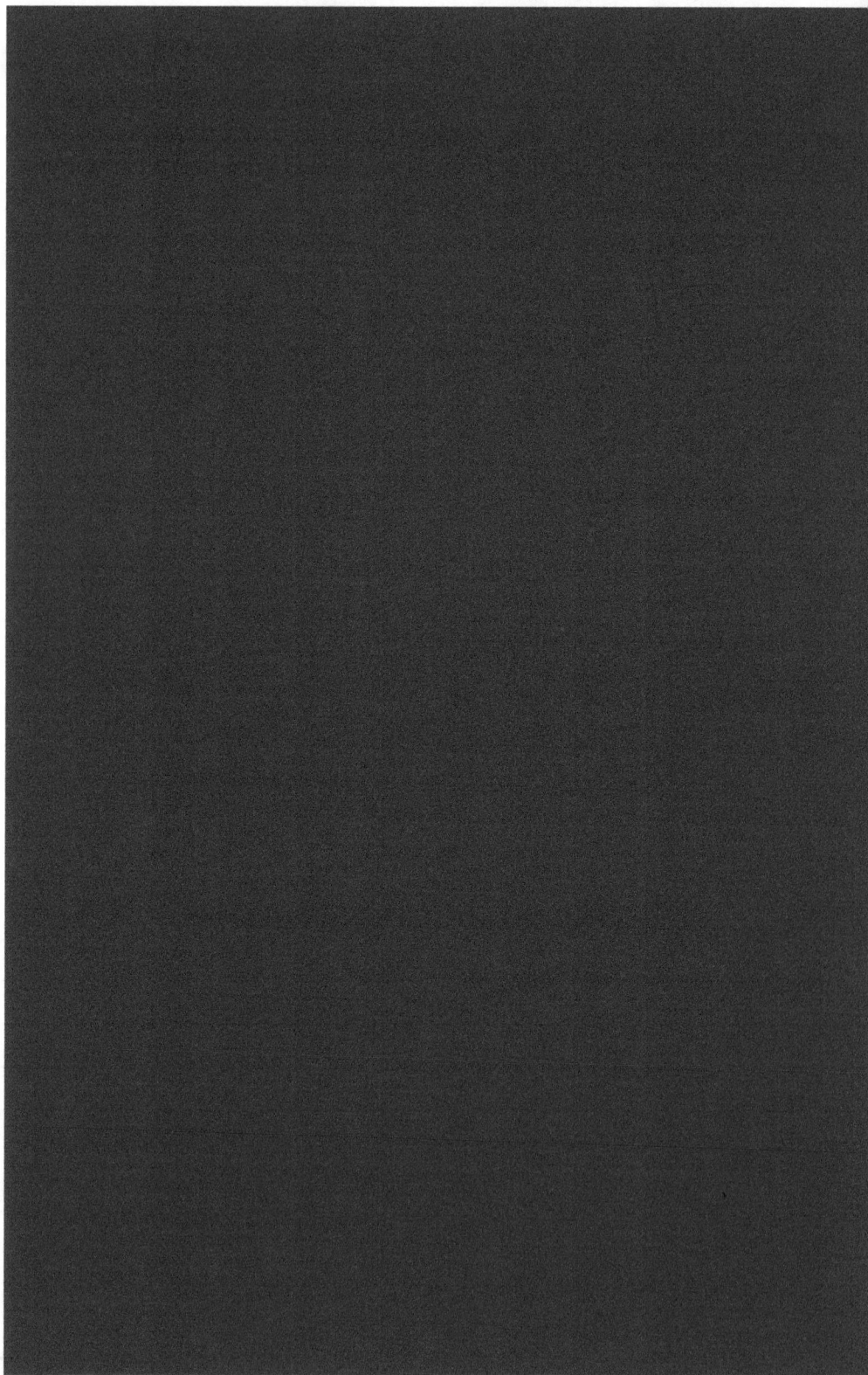

DATE   S M T W T F S

MORNING THOUGHTS & FEELINGS

_____
_____
_____
_____

MORNING MEAL @ _____

I ATE:
_____
_____

I DRANK:
_____

I FELT:
_____

2 3 HOURS LATER I FELT:
_____

MID MORNING SNACK @ _____

I ATE:
_____
_____

I DRANK:
_____

I FELT:
_____

AFTERNOON MEAL @ _____

I ATE:

_____
_____

I DRANK:

_____

I FELT:

_____

2-3 HOURS LATER I FELT:

_____

AFTERNOON SNACK @_____

I ATE:

_____
_____

I DRANK:

_____

I FELT:

_____

EVENING MEAL @_____

I ATE:

_____
_____

I DRANK:

_____

I FELT:

_____

2-3 HOURS LATER I FELT:

_____

HAPPINESS TRACKER - ON A SCALE OF 1-5

Rate the areas below from 1-5, with 1 being least happy & 5 being most happy. Pay close attention to any trends you begin to notice regarding how the things you eat & drink affect the way you feel & your overall happiness.

My morning energy level	○	○	○	○	○
My afternoon energy level	○	○	○	○	○
My evening energy level	○	○	○	○	○
How my body feels	○	○	○	○	○
My mental clarity	○	○	○	○	○
My emotional stability	○	○	○	○	○
My excitement about life	○	○	○	○	○
My personal relationships	○	○	○	○	○
My professional relationships	○	○	○	○	○
My poop	○	○	○	○	○

EVENING THOUGHTS & FEELINGS

_____

_____

_____

_____

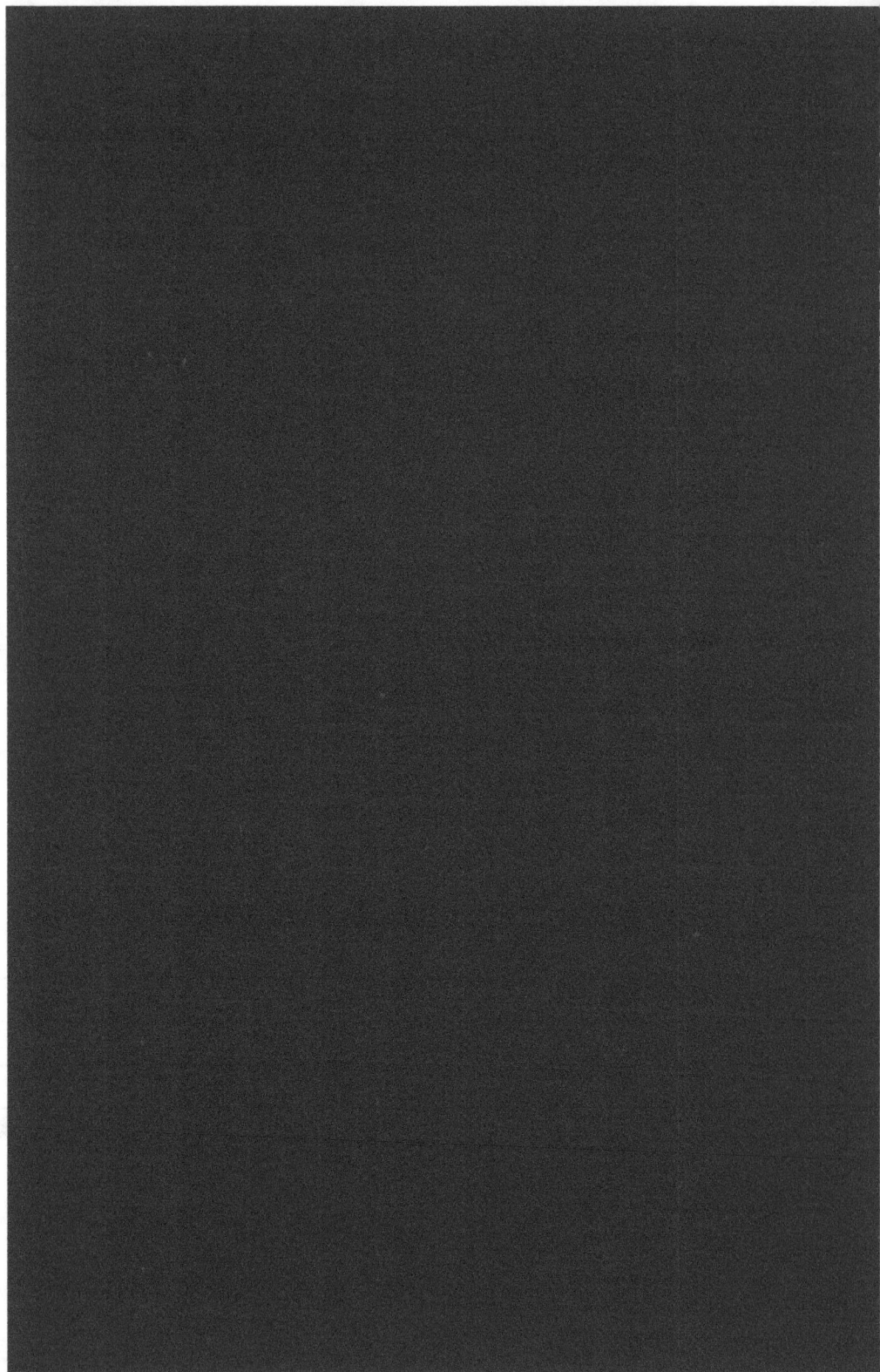

Day 41

DATE   S M T W T F S

MORNING THOUGHTS & FEELINGS

_____

_____

_____

_____

_____

MORNING MEAL @ _____

I ATE:

_____

_____

I DRANK:

_____

I FELT:

_____

2-3 HOURS LATER I FELT:

_____

MID MORNING SNACK @ _____

I ATE:

_____

_____

I DRANK:

_____

I FELT:

_____

AFTERNOON MEAL @ _____

I ATE:

_____
_____

I DRANK:

_____

I FELT:

_____

2-3 HOURS LATER I FELT:

_____

AFTERNOON SNACK @ _____

I ATE:

_____
_____

I DRANK:

_____

I FELT:

_____

EVENING MEAL @ _____

I ATE:

_____
_____

I DRANK:

_____

I FELT:

_____

2-3 HOURS LATER I FELT:

_____

HAPPINESS TRACKER - ON A SCALE OF 1-5

Rate the areas below from 1-5, with 1 being least happy & 5 being most happy. Pay close attention to any trends you begin to notice regarding how the things you eat & drink affect the way you feel & your overall happiness.

My morning energy level   ○ ○ ○ ○ ○

My afternoon energy level   ○ ○ ○ ○ ○

My evening energy level   ○ ○ ○ ○ ○

How my body feels   ○ ○ ○ ○ ○

My mental clarity   ○ ○ ○ ○ ○

My emotional stability   ○ ○ ○ ○ ○

My excitement about life   ○ ○ ○ ○ ○

My personal relationships   ○ ○ ○ ○ ○

My professional relationships   ○ ○ ○ ○ ○

My poop   ○ ○ ○ ○ ○

EVENING THOUGHTS & FEELINGS

_____

_____

_____

_____

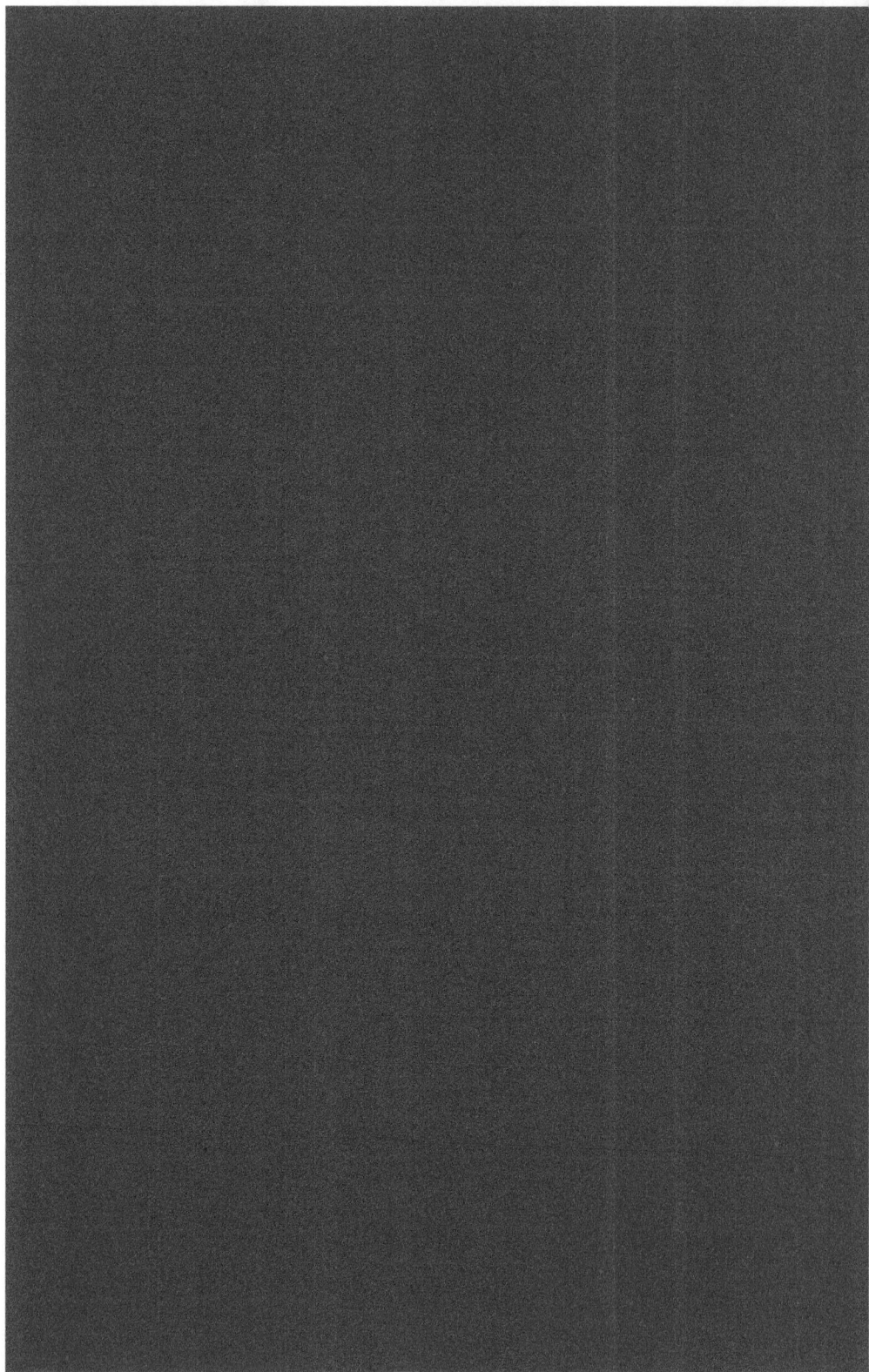

DATE _____   S M T W T F S

MORNING THOUGHTS & FEELINGS

_____

_____

_____

_____

MORNING MEAL @ _____

I ATE:

_____

_____

I DRANK:

_____

I FELT:

_____

2 3 HOURS LATER I FELT:

_____

MID MORNING SNACK @ _____

I ATE:

_____

_____

I DRANK:

_____

I FELT:

_____

AFTERNOON MEAL @ _____

I ATE:

_____
_____

I DRANK:

_____

I FELT:

_____

2-3 HOURS LATER I FELT:

_____

AFTERNOON SNACK @ _____

I ATE:

_____
_____

I DRANK:

_____

I FELT:

_____

EVENING MEAL @ _____

I ATE:

_____
_____
_____

I DRANK:

_____

I FELT:

_____

2-3 HOURS LATER I FELT:

_____

HAPPINESS TRACKER - ON A SCALE OF 1-5

Rate the areas below from 1-5, with 1 being least happy & 5 being most happy. Pay close attention to any trends you begin to notice regarding how the things you eat & drink affect the way you feel & your overall happiness.

My morning energy level   ○ ○ ○ ○ ○

My afternoon energy level   ○ ○ ○ ○ ○

My evening energy level   ○ ○ ○ ○ ○

How my body feels   ○ ○ ○ ○ ○

My mental clarity   ○ ○ ○ ○ ○

My emotional stability   ○ ○ ○ ○ ○

My excitement about life   ○ ○ ○ ○ ○

My personal relationships   ○ ○ ○ ○ ○

My professional relationships   ○ ○ ○ ○ ○

My poop   ○ ○ ○ ○ ○

EVENING THOUGHTS & FEELINGS

_____

_____

_____

_____

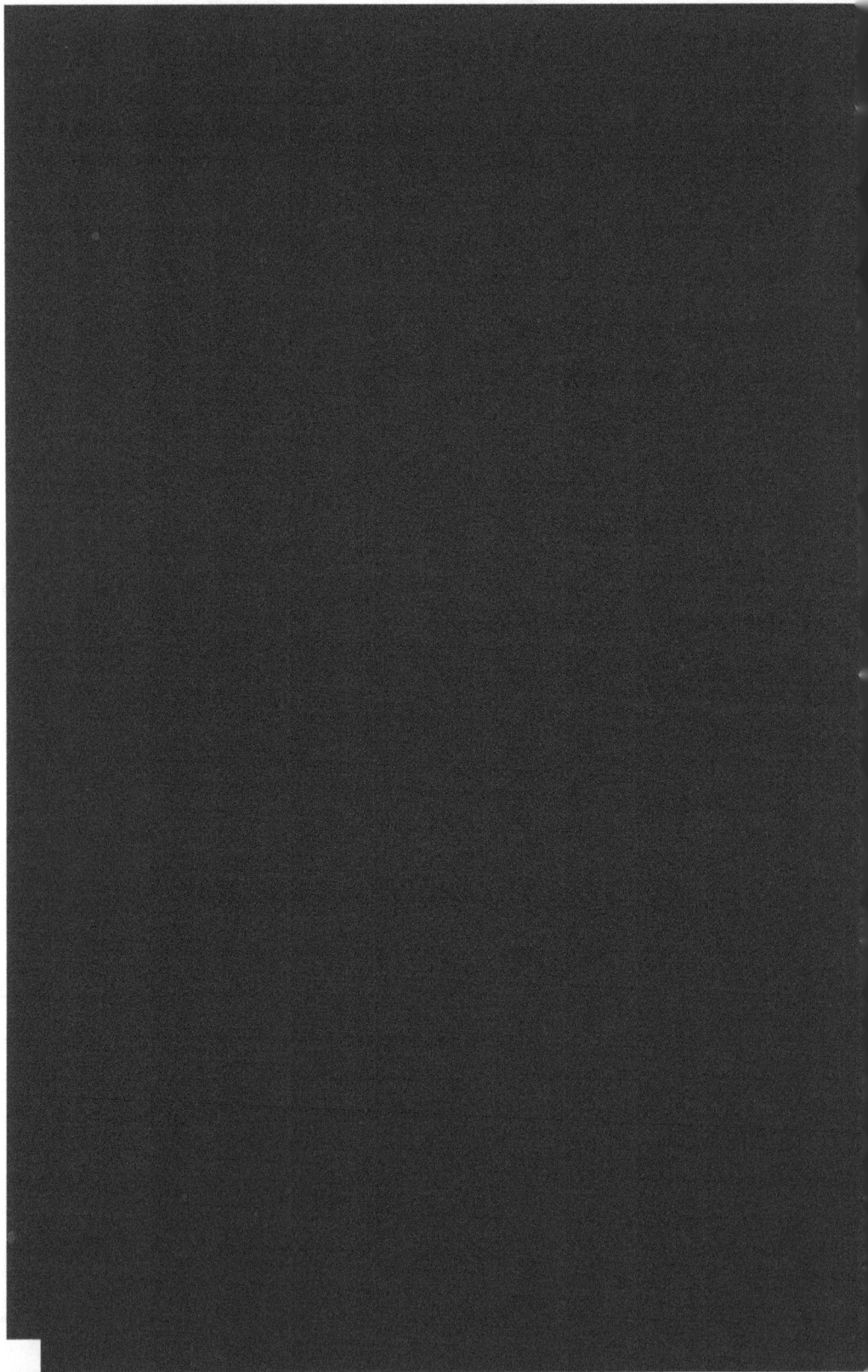

Well done!

You did it!

That's 6 weeks of tracking your thoughts, feelings, emotions, and eating habits. You're well on your way to developing a healthy and balance lifestyle by eating intuitively and listening to your body.

If you'd like to learn more about intuitive eating and what it looks like to work with a certified personal trainer 1:1 to develop your own unique fitness or nutrition plan, send me a message on Instagram @katzuanichwellness.

Be sure to follow me on Instagram for updates on future journals, trackers, and cookbooks.

About the Author

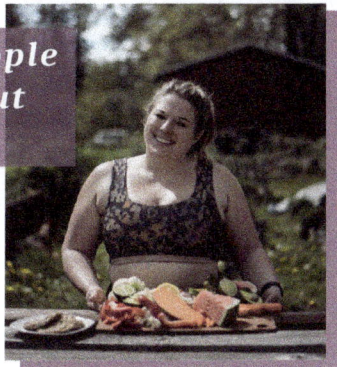

'My goal is to support & empower people to feel more love and less guilt about their lives, bodies & eating habits.'

Growing up in Bellingham, WA, Kat spent countless summers on the water salmon fishing with her dad & brothers who were commercial fishermen. This experience sparked a desire to have a clear understanding of where her food was coming from, as well as a drive to use fill her plate with fresh ingredients as often as possible.

After struggling with weight fluctuations, and an unhealthy relationship with food which often included deprivation and binge eating throughout her twenties, Kat knew that something needed to change. She set to work reclaiming her power over her relationships with food, herself, and how she viewed her body.

Kat began sharing this passion with others as a professional chef, caterer, and certified personal trainer, deepening her knowledge of nutrition, and strengthening her own health and life balance, while empowering others to do the same. She's currently studying for a Bachelor's degree in Health and Wellness Management at the University of Wisconsin.

'A healthy mindset, self-love, and acceptance can be the greatest tools for living a healthy life, which is the foundation of this journal. '

~ Kat

www.ingramcontent.com/pod-product-compliance
Lightning Source LLC
Chambersburg PA
CBHW070108030426
42335CB00016B/2063